T0331552

Computational Modeling of the COVID-19 Disease

Numerical ODE Analysis with R Programming

Computational Modeling of the COVID-19 Disease

Numerical ODE Analysis with R Programming

William E Schiesser

Lehigh University, USA

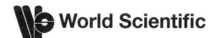
World Scientific

NEW JERSEY · LONDON · SINGAPORE · BEIJING · SHANGHAI · HONG KONG · TAIPEI · CHENNAI · TOKYO

Published by

World Scientific Publishing Co. Pte. Ltd.

5 Toh Tuck Link, Singapore 596224

USA office: 27 Warren Street, Suite 401-402, Hackensack, NJ 07601

UK office: 57 Shelton Street, Covent Garden, London WC2H 9HE

British Library Cataloguing-in-Publication Data

A catalogue record for this book is available from the British Library.

COMPUTATIONAL MODELING OF THE COVID-19 DISEASE
Numerical ODE Analysis with R Programming

ISBN 978-981-122-287-0 (hardcover)
ISBN 978-981-122-288-7 (ebook for institutions)
ISBN 978-981-122-289-4 (ebook for individuals)

For any available supplementary material, please visit
https://www.worldscientific.com/worldscibooks/10.1142/11899#t=suppl

Typeset by Stallion Press
Email: enquiries@stallionpress.com

Printed in Singapore

Contents

Preface   vii

Chapter 1.   Single Area ODE Model   1
(1)   Introduction   1
      (1.1)   USA model   1
      (1.1.1)   Susceptibles   1
      (1.1.2)   Asymptomatic infecteds   3
      (1.1.3)   Symptomatic infecteds   5
      (1.1.4)   Recovereds   6
      (1.1.5)   Deaths   7
      (1.2)   R routines   8
      (1.2.1)   Main program   9
      (1.2.2)   ODE routine   17
      (1.2.3)   Numerical, graphical output   21
      (1.2.4)   Parameter variation   24
      (1.3)   Summary and conclusions   29
References   29
Appendix A1   30

Chapter 2.   Detailed Analysis of the ODE Model   31
(2)   Introduction   31
      (2.1)   Time derviatives of the ODE model   31
      (2.1.1)   Main program   31

(2.1.2)   ODE routine   39
(2.1.3)   Numerical, graphical output   39
(2.1.4)   Analysis of ODE LHS, RHS terms   42
(2.2)   Summary and conclusions   58

Chapter 3.   Variants of the Basic ODE Model   61
(3)   Introduction   61
(3.1)   Limited susceptibles infection   61
(3.1.1)   Main program   63
(3.1.2)   ODE routine   64
(3.1.3)   Numerical, graphical output   66
(3.2)   Summary and conclusions   74

Chapter 4.   Postulated Vaccine/Therapeutic Drug
    Treatment   75
(4)   Introduction   75
(4.1)   ODE model with parameter time variation   75
(4.1.1)   Main program   76
(4.1.2)   ODE routine   77
(4.1.3)   Numerical, graphical output   79
(4.2)   Summary and conclusions   83

Chapter 5.   ODE Model with Delays   85
(5)   Introduction   85
(5.1)   ODE model with delays   85
(5.1.1)   Main program   86
(5.1.2)   ODE routine   87
(5.1.3)   Numerical, graphical output   90
(5.2)   Summary and conclusions   95
References   95

Index   97

Preface

This book presents a computer-based model for the dynamics of the COVID-19 epidemic that developed in late 2019. The model is an extension of the basic SIR (Susceptibles Infecteds Recovered) model and consists of five ordinary differential equations (ODEs) with the dependent variables:

$S(t)$ susceptible population

$I_a(t)$ asymptomatic infected population

$I_s(t)$ symptomatic infected population

$R(t)$ recovered population

$D(t)$ deaths

t time

The time scale in weeks is $0 \leq t \leq 52$ (one year), and the evolution of the five dependent variables is computed by the numerical integration of the five initial value ODEs from an initial condition (IC) of (1) the population for a country for $S(t = 0)$, (2) small values for $I_a(t = 0)$, $I_s(t = 0)$, and (3) zero values for $R(t = 0)$, $D(t = 0)$. $S(t)$ moves (2), (3) forward in time as an epidemic develops. The country selected is the United States (US) with $S(t = 0) = 3.3 \times 10^8$. Spatial variations within the country are not considered so that the ODE model is basic and introductory.

The numerical integration of the 5×5 (five equations in five unknowns) model is performed with routines coded (programmed) in R, a quality, open-source scientific computing system that is readily available from the Internet. Formal mathematics is minimized, e.g., no theorems and proofs. Rather, the presentation is through detailed examples that the reader/researcher/analyst can execute on modest computers. The five ODE dependent variables are plotted against t with basic R plotting utilities.

Chapter 1 is an introduction to the 5×5 ODE model with a detailed discussion of the associated R code. Chapter 2 presents a methodology for the computation and display of the ODE RHS terms and LHS derivatives in t. These terms explain the properties of the ODE solutions. Chapters 3,4 present variations of the basic ODE model, for example, (1) limitations on the rate of conversion of susceptibles to infecteds and (2) reductions in the rate of COVID-19 transmission resulting from a postulated vaccine or therapeutic drug. Chapter 5 concludes with a discussion of the ODEs that include selected rates delayed in time to reflect the incubation period of $I_a(t)$.

The routines are available from a download link so that the example models can be executed without having to first study numerical methods and computer coding. The routines can then be applied to variations and extensions of the ODE model, such as changes in the parameters and the form of the model equations.

The author would welcome comments/suggestions concerning this approach to the analysis of the COVID-19 epidemic (directed to wes1@lehigh.edu).

W. E. Schiesser
Bethlehem, PA, USA

Chapter 1

Single Area ODE Model

(1) Introduction

The numerical ordinary differential equation (ODE) analysis of the COVID-19[1] infectious disease starts with an extension of a basic SIR (Susceptible Infected Recovered) model. The SIR model is applied to a geographical area, generally a country. For the following discussion, the area is the United States.

(1.1) USA model

The SIR model is 5×5 (five ODEs in five unknowns) as explained next. The first ODE is a balance for the susceptible population, designated as $S(t)$. A basic assumption in stating this first equation is that the spatial variation of the susceptible population is not considered.

(1.1.1) Susceptibles

Eq. (1.1-1) defines $S(t)$.

$$\frac{dS}{dt} = r_p - r_{SI_a}SI_a - r_{SI_s}SI_s + r_R R \qquad (1.1\text{-}1)$$

---

[1]COVID-19 is the World Health Organization (WHO) designation for the coronavirus disease resulting in the pandemic starting in late 2019.

The RHS variables and parameters of eq. (1.1-1) are listed in Table 1.1.

S	susceptibles
I_a	asymptomatic infecteds
I_s	symptomatic infecteds
R	recovereds
t	time
r_p	susceptibles production rate
r_{SI_a}	susceptibles to asymptomatic infecteds rate constant
r_{SI_s}	susceptibles to symptomatic infecteds rate constant
r_R	return recovereds rate constant

Table 1.1: Variables and parameters of eq. (1.1-1)

Four populations are included in the ODE model, $S(t)$, $I_a(t)$, $I_s(t)$, $R(t)$. Two infected populations (infecteds) are included for asymptomatic infecteds (with no apparent symptoms of the COVID-19 infection), $I_a(t)$, and symptomatic infecteds (with recognizable symptoms of the COVID-19 infection), $I_s(t)$. The recovered population (recovereds), $R(t)$, is included to account for recovereds that revert back to susceptibles. The terms in eq. (1.1-1) are explained in more detail next.

- $\dfrac{dS}{dt}$: t derivative of susceptible population, $S(t)$. $\dfrac{dS}{dt} > 0$

for $S(t)$ increasing with t. $\dfrac{dS}{dt} < 0$ for $S(t)$ decreasing with t.

- r_p: Rate of increase of susceptible population with t from addition of susceptibles (e.g., from immigration, travel).

- $-r_{SI_a}SI_a$: Rate of decrease of susceptibles from asymptomatic infection. This is a nonlinear term (from the product SI_a) that accounts for the interaction of susceptibles and asymptomatic infecteds to define the rate of reduction of susceptibles from the transition to asymptomatic infecteds.

- $-r_{SI_s}SI_s$: Rate of decrease of susceptibles from symptomatic infection. This is a nonlinear term (from the product SI_s) that accounts for the interaction of susceptibles and symptomatic infecteds to define the rate of reduction of susceptibles from the transition to symptomatic infecteds.

- $+r_R R$: Rate of increase of susceptibles from recovereds that are reinfected.

Eq. (1.1-1) requires three additional ODEs that define $I_a(t), I_s(t), R(t)$.

(1.1.2) Asymptomatic infecteds

Eq. (1.1-2) defines $I_a(t)$.

$$\frac{dI_a}{dt} = r_{SI_a}SI_a - r_{I_sI_a}I_a - r_{RI_a}I_a - r_{DI_a}I_a \qquad (1.1\text{-}2)$$

The RHS variables and parameters of eq. (1.1-2) are listed in Table 1.2 (with some repetition of the terms in Table 1.1 so that the discussion of eq. (1.1-2) is self contained).

$$S \quad \text{susceptibles}$$

$$I_a \quad \text{asymptomatic infecteds}$$

$$I_s \quad \text{symptomatic infecteds}$$

$$t \quad \text{time}$$

r_{SI_a} susceptibles to asymptomatic infecteds
rate constant

$r_{I_aI_s}$ asymptomatic to symptomatic infecteds
rate constant

r_{RI_a} asymptotic infecteds to recovereds
rate constant

r_{DI_a} asymptomatic infecteds death
rate constant

Table 1.2: Variables and parameters of eq. (1.1-2)

The terms in eq. (1.1-2) are explained in more detail next.

- $\dfrac{dI_a}{dt}$: t derivative of asymptomatic infecteds population, $I_a(t)$. $\dfrac{dI_a}{dt} > 0$ for $I_a(t)$ increasing with t. $\dfrac{dI_a}{dt} < 0$ for $I_a(t)$ decreasing with t.
- $r_{SI_a}SI_a$: Rate of increase of asymptomatic infecteds from susceptibles. This is a nonlinear term (from the product SI_a).
- $-r_{I_sI_a}I_a$: Rate of decrease of asymptomatic infecteds from conversion to symptomatic infecteds.

- $-r_{RI_a}I_a$: Rate of decrease of asymptomatic infecteds from conversion to recovereds.
- $-r_{DI_a}I_a$: Death rate of asymptomatic infecteds.

(1.1.3) Symptomatic infecteds

Eq. (1.1-3) defines $I_s(t)$.

$$\frac{dI_s}{dt} = r_{SI_s}SI_s + r_{I_sI_a}I_a - r_{RI_s}I_s - r_{DI_s}I_s \qquad (1.1\text{-}3)$$

The RHS variables and parameters of eq. (1.1-3) are listed in Table 1.3 (with some repetition of the terms in Tables 1.1, 1.2 so that the discussion of eq. (1.1-3) is self contained).

S	susceptibles
I_s	symptomatic infecteds
I_a	asymptomatic infecteds
t	time
r_{SI_s}	susceptibles to symptomatic infecteds rate constant
$r_{I_aI_s}$	asymptomatic to symptomatic infecteds rate constant
r_{RI_a}	asymptomatic infecteds to recovereds rate constant
r_{DI_s}	symptomatic infecteds death rate constant

Table 1.3: Variables and parameters of eq. (1.1-3)

The terms in eq. (1.1-3) are explained in more detail next.

- $\dfrac{dI_s}{dt}$: t derivative of symptomatic infecteds population, $I_s(t)$. $\dfrac{dI_s}{dt} > 0$ for $I_s(t)$ increasing with t. $\dfrac{dI_s}{dt} < 0$ for $I_s(t)$ decreasing with t.
- $+r_{SI_s}SI_s$: Rate of increase of symptomatic infecteds from susceptibles. This is a nonlinear term (from the product SI_s).
- $+r_{I_sI_a}I_a$: Rate of increase of symptomatic infecteds from asymptomatic infecteds.
- $-r_{RI_s}I_s$ Rate of decrease of symptomatic infecteds to recovereds.
- $-r_{DI_s}I_s$: Death rate of symptomatic infecteds.

(1.1.4) Recovereds

Eq. (1.1-4) defines $R(t)$.

$$\frac{dR}{dt} = r_{RI_a}I_a + r_{RI_s}I_s - r_R R \tag{1.1-4}$$

The RHS variables and parameters of eq. (1.1-4) are listed in Table 1.4 (with some repetition of the terms in Tables 1.1 to 1.3 so that the discussion of eq. (1.1-4) is self contained).

The terms in eq. (1.1-4) are explained in more detail next.

- $\dfrac{dR}{dt}$: t derivative of recovereds population, $R(t)$. $\dfrac{dR}{dt} > 0$ for $R(t)$ increasing with t. $\dfrac{dR}{dt} < 0$ for $R(t)$ decreasing with t.
- $r_{RI_a}I_a$: Rate of increase of recovereds from asymptomatic infecteds.

- $+r_{RI_s}I_s$: Rate of increase of recoverids from symptomatic infecteds.
- $-r_R R$: Rate of recovereds returning to susceptible condition.

R	recovereds
I_a	asymptomatic infecteds
I_s	symptomatic infecteds
t	time
r_{RI_a}	asymptomatic infecteds to recovereds rate constant
r_{RI_s}	symptomatic infecteds to recovereds rate constant
r_R	return recovereds rate constant

Table 1.4: Variables and parameters of eq. (1.1-4)

(1.1.5) Deaths

Eq. (1.1-5) defines $D(t)$.

$$\frac{dD}{dt} = r_{DI_a}I_a + r_{DI_s}I_s \qquad (1.1\text{-}5)$$

The RHS variables and parameters of eq. (1.1-5) are listed in Table 1.5 (with some repetition of the terms in Tables 1.1 to 1.4 so that the discussion of eq. (1.1-5) is self contained).

D deaths

t time

r_{DI_a} asymptomatic infecteds death rate constant

r_{DI_s} symptomatic infecteds death rate constant

Table 1.5: Variables and parameters of eq. (1.1-5)

The terms in eq. (1.1-5) are explained in more detail next.

- $\dfrac{dD}{dt}$: t derivative of deaths, $D(t)$.
- $r_{DI_a}I_a$: Death rate from asymptomatic infecteds.
- $+r_{DI_s}I_s$: Death rate from symptomatic infecteds.

Eqs. (1.1) are first order in t and each requires an initial condition (IC).

$$S(t = 0) = S_0 \qquad\qquad (1.2\text{-}1)$$

$$I_a(t = 0) = I_{a0} \qquad\qquad (1.2\text{-}2)$$

$$I_s(t = 0) = I_{s0} \qquad\qquad (1.2\text{-}3)$$

$$R(t = 0) = R_0 \qquad\qquad (1.2\text{-}4)$$

$$D(t = 0) = D_0 \qquad\qquad (1.2\text{-}5)$$

$S_0, I_{a0}, I_{s0}, R_0, D_0$ are constants to be specified.

This completes the statement of the ODE/SIR model (eqs. (1.1), (1.2)). A set of R routines for the implmentation of this model is considered next.

(1.2) R routines

The R routines that implement eqs. (1.1), (1.2) follow.

(1.2.1) Main program

A main program for eqs. (1.1) is in Listing 1.1.

```
#
# COV model
#
# Delete previous workspaces
  rm(list=ls(all=TRUE))
#
# Access DODE integrator
  library(deSolve)
#
# Access functions for numerical solution
  setwd("f:/cov/chap1");
  source("ode1a.R");
#
# Model parameters
#
# S(t)
  rp=0.001;
  rSIa=1;
  rSIs=1;
  rR=0.001;
  Stot=3.3e+08;
#
# Ia(t)
#
# Is(t)
  rIsIa=0.1;
#
# R(t)
  rRIa=0.5;
  rRIs=0.5;
#
```

```
# D(t)
  rDIa=0.001;
  rDIs=0.001;
#
# Temporal grid
  nout=51;t0=0;tf=52;
  tout=seq(from=t0,to=tf,by=(tf-t0)/(nout-1));
#
# IC vector
  y0=rep(0,5);
   S0=1; y0[1]= S0;
  Ia0=1.0e-06; y0[2]=Ia0;
  Is0=1.0e-07; y0[3]=Is0;
   R0=0; y0[4]= R0;
   D0=0; y0[5]= D0;
  ncall=0;
#
# ODE integration
  out=lsodes(y=y0,times=tout,func=ode1a,
      sparsetype ="sparseint",rtol=1e-6,
      atol=1e-6,maxord=5);
  nrow(out)
  ncol(out)
#
# Arrays/vectors for ODE solutions
   Sp=rep(0,nout);
  Iap=rep(0,nout);
  Isp=rep(0,nout);
   Rp=rep(0,nout);
   Dp=rep(0,nout);
   tp=rep(0,nout);
  for(it in 1:nout){
    tp[it]=out[it,1];
    Sp[it]=out[it,2]*Stot;
```

```
    Iap[it]=out[it,3]*Stot;
    Isp[it]=out[it,4]*Stot;
     Rp[it]=out[it,5]*Stot;
     Dp[it]=out[it,6]*Stot;
   }
#
# Display numerical solution
  iv=seq(from=1,to=nout,by=10);
  for(it in iv){
    cat(sprintf("\n                t"));
    cat(sprintf("\n%12.1f\n",tp[it]));
    cat(sprintf("         S(t)            Ia(t)
                Is(t)"));
    cat(sprintf("\n           R(t)            D(t)
                sum"));
    cat(sprintf("\n%12.2e %12.2e %12.2e",
                Sp[it],Iap[it],Isp[it]));
    sum=Sp[it]+Iap[it]+Isp[it]+Rp[it]+Dp[it];
    cat(sprintf("\n%12.2e%13.2e%13.2e\n",
                Rp[it],Dp[it],sum));
  }
#
# Display calls to pde1a
  cat(sprintf("\n ncall = %4d\n",ncall));
#
# 3 (rows) x 2 (columns) matrix
  par(mfrow=c(3,2));
#
# Plot ODE dependent variables
  plot(tp,Sp,type="l",xlab="t (wk)",ylab="S(t)",
       lty=1,main="S(t)",lwd=2,col="black");
  plot(tp,Iap,type="l",xlab="t (wk)",ylab="Ia(t)",
       lty=1,main="Ia(t)",lwd=2,col="black");
  plot(tp,Isp,type="l",xlab="t (wk)",ylab="Is(t)",
```

```
        lty=1,main="Is(t)",lwd=2,col="black");
plot(tp,Rp,type="l",xlab="t (wk)",ylab="R(t)",
        lty=1,main="R(t)",lwd=2,col="black");
plot(tp,Dp,type="l",xlab="t (wk)",ylab="D(t)",
        lty=1,main="D(t)",lwd=2,col="black");
plot(tp,Sp+Iap+Isp+Rp+Dp,type="l",xlab="t (wk)",
        ylab="sum",lty=1,main="sum",lwd=2,
        col="black");
```

Listing 1.1: Main program for eqs. (1.1), (1.2)

We can note the following details about the main program of Listing 1.1.

- Previous workspaces are deleted.

```
#
# COV model
#
# Delete previous workspaces
  rm(list=ls(all=TRUE))
```

- The R ODE integrator library deSolve is accessed. Then the directory with the files for the solution of eqs. (1.1) is designated. Note that setwd (set working directory) uses / rather than the usual \.

```
#
# Access DODE integrator
  library(deSolve)
#
# Access functions for numerical solution
  setwd("f:/cov/chap1");
  source("ode1a.R");
```

ode1a.R is the routine with the programming of eqs. (1.1).

- The model parameters are specified numerically.

```
#
# Model parameters
#
# S(t)
  rp=0.001;
  rSIa=1;
  rSIs=1;
  rR=0.001;
  Stot=3.3e+08;
#
# Ia(t)
#
# Is(t)
  rIsIa=0.1;
#
# R(t)
  rRIa=0.5;
  rRIs=0.5;
#
# D(t)
  rDIa=0.001;
  rDIs=0.001;
```

The parameter values were selected to give a time scale of 52 wks (weeks) as explained subsequently. For $S(t)$ defined by eq. (1.1-1), the total population is Stot=3.3e+08 (3.3×10^8 susceptibles), the population of the United States (US) in 2019.

For $I_a(t)$ defined by eq. (1.1-2), the parameters are specified for $S(t), I_s(t)$ and used for $I_a(t)$ as well.

- An interval in t of 51 points is defined for $0 \leq t \leq 52$ wks so that tout=0,52/50,...,52.

```
#
# Temporal grid
  nout=51;t0=0;tf=52;
  tout=seq(from=t0,to=tf,by=(tf-t0)/(nout-1));
```

- The ICs of eqs. (1.2) are defined in a vector y0.

```
#
# IC vector
  y0=rep(0,5);
   S0=1; y0[1]= S0;
  Ia0=1.0e-06; y0[2]=Ia0;
  Is0=1.0e-07; y0[3]=Is0;
   R0=0; y0[4]= R0;
   D0=0; y0[5]= D0;
  ncall=0;
```

$S(t = 0) = 1$ so that the initial susceptible population is normalized to one. Relative to this normalized susceptible population, the other four ICs are $I_a(t = 0) = 1.0 \times 10^{-6}$, $I_s(t = 0) = 1.0 \times 10^{-7}$, $R(t = 0) = 0$, $D(t = 0) = 0$. Of particular interest is how the susceptible population moves the other four dependent variables away from the initial values (through the numerical integration of eqs. (1.1)).

Also, the counter for the calls to ode1a is initialized.

- The system of 5 ODEs is integrated by the library integrator lsodes (available in deSolve, [1]). As expected, the inputs to lsodes are the ODE function, ode1a, the IC vector y0, and the vector of output values of t, tout. The length of y0 (5) informs lsodes how many ODEs are to be integrated. func,y,times are reserved names.

```
#
# ODE integration
  out=lsodes(y=y0,times=tout,func=ode1a,
```

```
    sparsetype ="sparseint",rtol=1e-6,
    atol=1e-6,maxord=5);
  nrow(out)
  ncol(out)
```

The numerical solution to the ODEs is returned in matrix out. In this case, out has the dimensions nout $\times$ $(5+1) = 51 \times 6$, which are confirmed by the output from nrow(out),ncol(out) (included in the numerical output considered subsequently). The offset $+1$ is required since the first element of out is the value of t, and the 2 to 6 elements are the values of $S(t), I_a(t), I_s(t), R(t), D(t)$.

- Vectors are defined for the computed ODE solution (in array out returned by lsodes). The solution is then placed in these arrays.

```
#
# Arrays/vectors for ODE solutions
   Sp=rep(0,nout);
  Iap=rep(0,nout);
  Isp=rep(0,nout);
   Rp=rep(0,nout);
   Dp=rep(0,nout);
   tp=rep(0,nout);
  for(it in 1:nout){
    tp[it]=out[it,1];
    Sp[it]=out[it,2]*Stot;
   Iap[it]=out[it,3]*Stot;
   Isp[it]=out[it,4]*Stot;
    Rp[it]=out[it,5]*Stot;
    Dp[it]=out[it,6]*Stot;
  }
```

Again, the offset $+1$ is required since the first element of each solution vector (for a particular index it) is the value of t associated with the solution.

The susceptible population, `Stot = 3.3e+08`, is used to scale the normalized populations to values that then can be compared with observed values.

- The five dependent variables $S(t), I_a(t), I_s(t), R(t), D(t)$ are displayed as a function of t with a `for`. Every tenth value of t appears from `by=10`.

```
#
# Display numerical solution
  iv=seq(from=1,to=nout,by=10);
  for(it in iv){
    cat(sprintf("\n                  t"));
    cat(sprintf("\n%12.1f\n",tp[it]));
    cat(sprintf("         S(t)            Ia(t)
                 Is(t)"));
    cat(sprintf("\n          R(t)              D(t)
                 sum"));
    cat(sprintf("\n%12.2e %12.2e %12.2e",
                 Sp[it],Iap[it],Isp[it]));
    sum=Sp[it]+Iap[it]+Isp[it]+Rp[it]+Dp[it];
    cat(sprintf("\n%12.2e%13.2e%13.2e\n",
                 Rp[it],Dp[it],sum));
  }
```

The sum of the five dependent variables is also computed and displayed, which is an important check of the model and coding as explained subsequently.

- The number of calls to `ode1a` is displayed at the end of the solution.

```
#
# Display calls to pde1a
  cat(sprintf("\n ncall = %4d\n",ncall));
```

- The five dependent variables are plotted against t with the R utility `plot`. The argument `type="l"` specifies a continuous line (rather than discrete points).

```
#
# 3 (rows) x 2 (columns) matrix
  par(mfrow=c(3,2));
#
# Plot ODE dependent variables
plot(tp,Sp,type="l",xlab="t(wk)",ylab="S(t)",
        lty=1,main="S(t)",lwd=2,col="black");
plot(tp,Iap,type="l",xlab="t(wk)",ylab="Ia(t)",
        lty=1,main="Ia(t)",lwd=2,col="black");
plot(tp,Isp,type="l",xlab="t(wk)",ylab="Is(t)",
        lty=1,main="Is(t)",lwd=2,col="black");
plot(tp,Rp,type="l",xlab="t(wk)",ylab="R(t)",
        lty=1,main="R(t)",lwd=2,col="black");
plot(tp,Dp,type="l",xlab="t(wk)",ylab="D(t)",
        lty=1,main="D(t)",lwd=2,col="black");
plot(tp,Sp+Iap+Isp+Rp+Dp,type="l",xlab="t(wk)",
        ylab="sum",lty=1,main="sum",lwd=2,
        col="black");
```

With `par(mfrow=c(3,2));`, the five dependent variables $S(t), I_a(t), I_s(t), R(t), D(t)$ are placed in a 3 rows $\times$ 2 columns matrix on one page (Fig. 1.1 considered subsequently). The sum of the five populations is also plotted.

This completes the discussion of the main program of Listing 1.1. The subordinate routine `ode1a` called by ODE integrator `lsodes` is considered next.

(1.2.2) ODE routine

`ode1a` follows in Listing 1.2.

```
ode1a=function(t,y,parm) {
#
# Function ode1a computes the t derivative
# vectors of S(t),Ia(t),Is(t),R(t),D(t)
#
# One vector to five scalars
   S=y[1];
  Ia=y[2];
  Is=y[3];
   R=y[4];
   D=y[5];
#
# ODEs
   St=rp-rSIa*S*Ia-rSIs*S*Is+rR*R;
   Iat=rSIa*S*Ia-rIsIa*Ia-
      rRIa*Ia-rDIa*Ia;
   Ist=rSIs*S*Is+rIsIa*Ia-
      rRIs*Is-rDIs*Is;
   Rt=rRIa*Ia+rRIs*Is-rR*R;
   Dt=rDIa*Ia+rDIs*Is;
#
# Five scalars to one vector
  yt=rep(0,5);
  yt[1]=St;
  yt[2]=Iat;
  yt[3]=Ist;
  yt[4]=Rt;
  yt[5]=Dt;
#
# Increment calls to ncall
  ncall <<- ncall+1;
#
# Return ODE t vector
  return(list(c(yt)));
```

```
#
# End of ode1a
  }
```

Listing 1.2: ODE routine ode1a for eqs. (1.1)

We can note the following details about the ODE programming of Listing 1.2.

- The function is defined.

```
  ode1a=function(t,y,parm) {
#
# Function ode1a computes the t derivative
# vectors of S(t),Ia(t),Is(t),R(t),D(t)
```

  t is the current value of t in eqs. (1.1). y is the 5-vector of ODE dependent variables. parm is an argument to pass parameters to ode1a (unused, but required in the argument list). The arguments must be listed in the order stated to properly interface with lsodes called in the main program of Listing 1.1. The derivative vector of the LHS of eqs. (1.1) is calculated and returned to lsodes as explained subsequently.
- Vector y is placed in five scalars to facilitate the programming of eqs. (1.1).

```
#
# One vector to five scalars
    S=y[1];
    Ia=y[2];
    Is=y[3];
    R=y[4];
    D=y[5];
```

- Eq. (1.1-1) is programmed ($\texttt{St} = \dfrac{dS}{dt}$).

```
#
# ODEs
  St=rp-rSIa*S*Ia-rSIs*S*Is+rR*R;
```

The parameters (constants) defined in the main program of Listing 1.1 are available to **ode1a** without any special designation (a feature of R).

- Eq. (1.1-2) is programmed ($\texttt{Iat} = \dfrac{dI_a}{dt}$).

```
  Iat=rSIa*S*Ia-rIsIa*Ia-
      rRIa*Ia-rDIa*Ia;
```

Lines can be continued onto second lines without any special designation (a feature of R), but a character at the end of the first line indicating a continuation is recommended, e.g., the first line ends in – indicating a continuation onto a second line. This is a better procedure than placing the – at the beginning of the second line.

- Eq. (1.1-3) is programmed ($\texttt{Ist} = \dfrac{dI_s}{dt}$).

```
  Ist=rSIs*S*Is+rIsIa*Ia-
      rRIs*Is-rDIs*Is;
```

- Eq. (1.1-4) is programmed ($\texttt{Rt} = \dfrac{dR}{dt}$).

```
  Rt=rRIa*Ia+rRIs*Is-rR*R;
```

- Eq. (1.1-5) is programmed ($\texttt{Dt} = \dfrac{dD}{dt}$).

```
  Dt=rDIa*Ia+rDIs*Is;
```

- With the completion of the five LHS t derivatives of eqs. (1.1), the derivatives are placed in a vector **yt** for return to **lsodes**.

```
#
# Five scalars to one vector
  yt=rep(0,5);
  yt[1]=St;
  yt[2]=Iat;
  yt[3]=Ist
  yt[4]=Rt;
  yt[5]=Dt;
```

- The counter for the calls to ode1a is incremented and returned to the main program of Listing 1.1 by <<-.

```
#
# Increment calls to ncall
  ncall <<- ncall+1;
```

- The vector yt is returned to lsodes for the next step along the solution.

```
#
# Return ODE t vector
  return(list(c(yt)));
#
# End of ode1a
  }
```

The vector yt is returned as a list as required by lsodes. c is the R vector utility. The final } concludes ode1a.

This completes the discussion of ode1a. The output from the main program of Listing 1.1 and ODE routine ode1a of Listing 1.2 is considered next.

(1.2.3) Numerical, graphical output

The numerical output is in Table 1.6.

[1] 51

[1] 6

```
            t
          0.0
        S(t)            Ia(t)            Is(t)
        R(t)             D(t)             sum
    3.30e+08         3.30e+02         3.30e+01
    0.00e+00         0.00e+00         3.30e+08


            t
         10.4
        S(t)            Ia(t)            Is(t)
        R(t)             D(t)             sum
    3.33e+08         3.04e+04         9.31e+04
    1.21e+05         2.43e+02         3.33e+08


            t
         20.8
        S(t)            Ia(t)            Is(t)
        R(t)             D(t)             sum
    2.95e+08         1.74e+06         1.83e+07
    2.21e+07         4.43e+04         3.37e+08


            t
         31.2
        S(t)            Ia(t)            Is(t)
        R(t)             D(t)             sum
    8.47e+07         7.02e+05         2.22e+07
    2.32e+08         4.67e+05         3.40e+08


            t
         41.6
        S(t)            Ia(t)            Is(t)
```

R(t)	D(t)	sum
7.21e+07	1.41e+04	1.28e+06
2.70e+08	5.48e+05	3.44e+08

t
52.0

S(t)	Ia(t)	Is(t)
R(t)	D(t)	sum
7.74e+07	2.93e+02	7.42e+04
2.69e+08	5.52e+05	3.47e+08

ncall =   135

Table 1.6: Numerical output from Listings 1.1, 1.2

We can note the following details about this output.

- 51 t output points as the first dimension of the solution matrix out from lsodes as programmed in the main program of Listing 1.1 (with nout=51).
- The solution matrix out returned by lsodes has 6 elements as a second dimension. The first element is the value of t. Elements 2 to 6 are $S(t), Ia(t), Is(t), R(t), D(t)$ from eqs. (1.1) (for each of the 51 output points).
- The solution is displayed for t=0, 52*10/50=10.4,..., 52 as programmed in Listing 1.1 (every tenth value of t is displayed as explained previously).
- ICs (1.2) are confirmed ($t = 0$).
- $S(t), Ia(t), Is(t), R(t), D(t)$ sum to a near constant value in t, starting with $S(t = 0) = 3.3 \times 10^8$. This is an important test of eqs. (1.1) as discussed in the chapter Appendix A1.
- The deaths, $D(t)$, are about $1/500$ of the recoverds, $R(t)$. For example, at $t = 52$, $D(t = 52)/R(t = 52) = 5.52 \times 10^5/2.69 \times 10^8 = 0.002052 \approx 1/500$. This level

of deaths relative to recovereds is investigated subsequently by varying the transmission rate constants in eqs. (1.1-1,2,3), r_{SI_a} (= rSIa in Listing 1.1), r_{SI_s} (= rSIs in Listing 1.1).

- The computational effort as indicated by ncall = 135 is modest so that lsodes computed the solution to eqs. (1.1) efficiently.

The graphical output is in Fig. 1.1.

The solutions $S(t), Ia(t), Is(t), R(t), D(t)$ approach a steady state. The sum of the five dependent variables, sum, has a small increase with t that is the result of the susceptible production term in eq. (1.1), r_p as explained in Appendix A1.

(1.2.4) Parameter variation

The solution in Table 1.6 and Fig. 1.1 can be considered as a base case of the model of eqs. (1.1), (1.2), and the effect of changes of the parameters defined numerically in Listing 1.1 can now be studied. For example, the transmission rate constants can be changed from

```
#
# S(t)
  rp=0.001;
  rSIa=1;
  rSIs=1;
```

to

```
#
# S(t)
  rp=0.001;
  rSIa=0.5;
  rSIs=0.5;
```

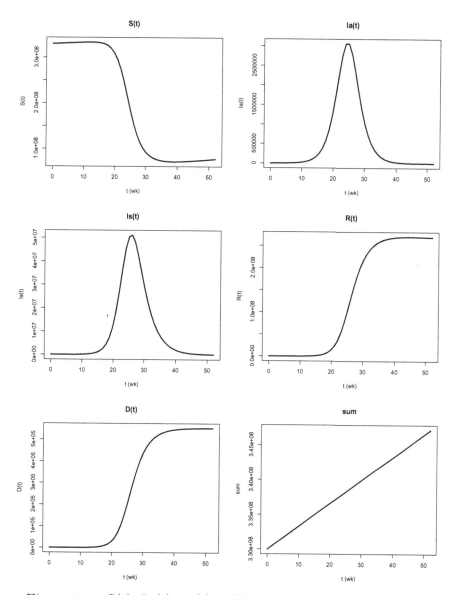

Figure 1.1: $S(t), Ia(t), Is(t), R(t), D(t)$ from eqs. (1.1), (1.2)

to represent the effect of a vaccine or antiviral therapeutic drug. The solution is summarized in Table 1.7 and Fig. 1.2.

```
[1] 51

[1] 6
              t
            0.0
          S(t)            Ia(t)            Is(t)
          R(t)            D(t)             sum
      3.30e+08        3.30e+02         3.30e+01
      0.00e+00        0.00e+00         3.30e+08


              t
           10.4
          S(t)            Ia(t)            Is(t)
          R(t)            D(t)             sum
      3.33e+08        1.25e+02         2.45e+02
      1.89e+03        3.80e+00         3.33e+08


              t
           20.8
          S(t)            Ia(t)            Is(t)
          R(t)            D(t)             sum
      3.37e+08        4.96e+01         3.49e+02
      3.85e+03        7.79e+00         3.37e+08


              t
           31.2
          S(t)            Ia(t)            Is(t)
          R(t)            D(t)             sum
      3.40e+08        2.07e+01         4.32e+02
      6.02e+03        1.22e+01         3.40e+08
```

```
        t
      41.6
      S(t)           Ia(t)           Is(t)
      R(t)           D(t)            sum
   3.44e+08       8.86e+00        5.33e+02
   8.52e+03       1.74e+01        3.44e+08


        t
      52.0
      S(t)           Ia(t)           Is(t)
      R(t)           D(t)            sum
   3.47e+08       3.94e+00        6.81e+02
   1.16e+04       2.37e+01        3.47e+08


ncall =    64
```

Table 1.7: Numerical output from Listings 1.1, 1.2,
rSIa=rSIs=0.5

A comparison of Tables 1.6 and 1.7, and Figs. 1.1 and 1.2, indicates the change from rSIa=rSIs=1 to rSIa=rSIs=0.5 essentially avoids the epidemic/pandemic.

For example, Table 1.7 indicates that the recovereds and deaths are small. The following summary at $t = 52$ wks indicates the differences in the solutions.

```
Table 1.6, rSIa = rSIs = 1

        t
      52.0
      S(t)           Ia(t)           Is(t)
      R(t)           D(t)            sum
   7.74e+07       2.93e+02        7.42e+04
   2.69e+08       5.52e+05        3.47e+08
```

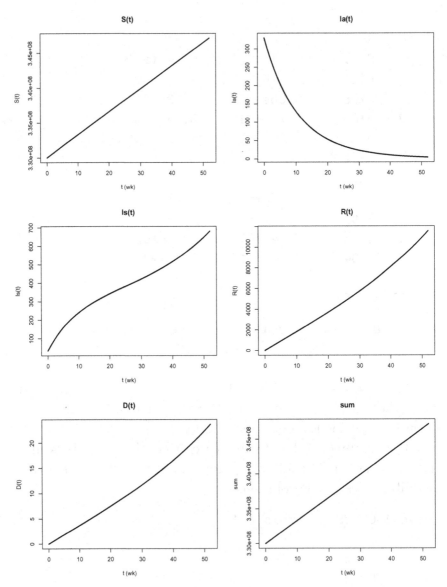

Figure 1.2: $S(t), Ia(t), Is(t), R(t), D(t)$ from eqs. (1.1), (1.2), rSIa=rSIs=0.5

```
Table 1.7, rSIa = rSIs = 0.5

        t
      52.0
      S(t)          Ia(t)          Is(t)
      R(t)          D(t)           sum
    3.47e+08      3.94e+00       6.81e+02
    1.16e+04      2.37e+01       3.47e+08
```

The deaths are changed from 5.52e+05 = 552,000 to 23.7. Clearly, rSia, rSis are very sensitive parameters. In summary, the postulated effect of a vaccine or antiviral drug can be a major reduction in deaths, and this conclusion is based on a small decrease in the transmission rate constants (1 to 0.5).

(1.3) Summary and conclusions

A basic 3 × 3 SIR ODE model is extended by including two infected states (dependent variables for asymptomatic and symptomatic populations) and an ODE for deaths. The R routines for the resulting a 5 × 5 basic ODE model is discussed initially, with the solutions presented in Table 1.6 and Fig. 1.1. Variation in parameter values is then demonstrated by reducing the transmission rate constants and analyzing the changes in the ODE model solution.

The origin of the factors that forestall the epidemic/ pandemic are considered in Chapter 2. Obviously this reduction did not occur, since, for example, a vaccine or effective therapeutic drug was not available when the coronavirus first appeared.

References

[1] Soetaert, K., J. Cash, and F. Mazzia (2012), *Solving Differential Equations in R*, Springer-Verlag, Heidelberg, Germany.

Appendix A1

Eqs. (1.1) follow a conservation principle for the total population that is demonstrated by adding the five ODEs.

$$\frac{dS}{dt} + \frac{dI_a}{dt} + \frac{dI_s}{dt} + \frac{dR}{dt} + \frac{dD}{dt} =$$

$$r_p - r_{SI_a}SI_a - r_{SI_s}SI_s + r_R R$$

$$+ (r_{SI_a}SI_a - r_{I_sI_a}I_a - r_{RI_a}I_a - r_{DI_a}I_a)$$

$$+ (r_{SI_s}SI_s + r_{I_sI_a}I_a - r_{RI_s}I_s - r_{DI_s}I_s)$$

$$+ (r_{RI_a}I_a + r_{RI_s}I_s - r_R R)$$

$$+ (r_{DI_a}I_a + r_{DI_s}I_s)$$

or

$$\frac{d\left(S + I_a + I_s + R + D\right)}{dt} = r_p \qquad \text{(A1.1-1)}$$

Eq. (A1.1-1) indicates that the sum of the five ODE dependent variables increases linearly in t with a slope r_p. This linear variation is demonstrated in the $sum(t)$ against t plot in Fig. 1.1 for $r_p = 0.001$ (defined in Listing 1.1). If $r_p = 0$ (no change in the total US population), the sum would not vary with t. Confirmation of this case is left as an exercise.

The special case

$$\frac{d\ sum}{dt} = r_p \qquad \text{(A1.1-2)}$$

is an important check of the ODE model (eqs. (1.1)) and the associated coding in ode1a of Listing 1.2. A departure from eq. (A1.1-2) would indicate an error in the model equations and/or the programming.

Chapter 2

Detailed Analysis of the ODE Model

(2) Introduction

The integration of the 5×5 ordinary differential equation (ODE) model presented in Chapter 1 gives the numerical solution $S(t), I_a(t), I_s(t), R(t), D(t)$. The origin of the features of these solutions is considered next.

(2.1) Time derviatives of the ODE model

The characteristics of the solutions $S(t), I_a(t), I_s(t), R(t), D(t)$ follow from the integration of the derivatives $\dfrac{dS(t)}{dt}, \dfrac{dI_a(t)}{dt}, \dfrac{dI_s(t)}{dt}, \dfrac{dR(t)}{dt}, \dfrac{dD(t)}{dt}$, that is, the LHSs of eqs. (1.1). Once the solutions are available, they can be used to calculate and display the derivatives.

(2.1.1) Main program

The main program of Listing 2.1 is an extension of the main program of Listing 1.1 with calculation and display of the derivative vector added at the end.

```
#
# COV model
#
# Delete previous workspaces
```

```
  rm(list=ls(all=TRUE))
#
# Access DODE integrator
  library(deSolve)
#
# Access functions for numerical solution
  setwd("f:/cov/chap2");
  source("ode1a.R");
#
# Model parameters
#
# S(t)
  rp=0.001;
  rSIa=1;
  rSIs=1;
  rR=0.001;
  Stot=3.3e+08;
#
# Ia(t)
#
# Is(t)
  rIsIa=0.1;
#
# R(t)
  rRIa=0.5;
  rRIs=0.5;
#
# D(t)
  rDIa=0.001;
  rDIs=0.001;
#
# Temporal grid
  nout=51;t0=0;tf=52;
  tout=seq(from=t0,to=tf,by=(tf-t0)/(nout-1));
```

```
#
# IC vector
  y0=rep(0,5);
   S0=1; y0[1]= S0;
  Ia0=1.0e-06; y0[2]=Ia0;
  Is0=1.0e-07; y0[3]=Is0;
   R0=0; y0[4]= R0;
   D0=0; y0[5]= D0;
  ncall=0;
#
# ODE integration
  nre=1;
  out=lsodes(y=y0,times=tout,func=ode1a,
      sparsetype ="sparseint",rtol=1e-6,
      atol=1e-6,maxord=5);
  nrow(out)
  ncol(out)
#
# Arrays/vectors for ODE solutions
   Sp=rep(0,nout);
  Iap=rep(0,nout);
  Isp=rep(0,nout);
   Rp=rep(0,nout);
   Dp=rep(0,nout);
   tp=rep(0,nout);
  for(it in 1:nout){
    tp[it]=out[it,1];
    Sp[it]=out[it,2]*Stot;
   Iap[it]=out[it,3]*Stot;
   Isp[it]=out[it,4]*Stot;
    Rp[it]=out[it,5]*Stot;
    Dp[it]=out[it,6]*Stot;
  }
#
```

```
# Display numerical solution
  iv=seq(from=1,to=nout,by=10);
  for(it in iv){
    cat(sprintf("\n                t"));
    cat(sprintf("\n%12.1f\n",tp[it]));
    cat(sprintf("          S(t)           Ia(t)
                  Is(t)"));
    cat(sprintf("\n          R(t)           D(t)
                  sum"));
    cat(sprintf("\n%12.2e %12.2e %12.2e",
                Sp[it],Iap[it],Isp[it]));
    sum=Sp[it]+Iap[it]+Isp[it]+Rp[it]+Dp[it];
    cat(sprintf("\n%12.2e%13.2e%13.2e\n",
                Rp[it],Dp[it],sum));
  }
#
# Display calls to pde1a
  cat(sprintf("\n ncall = %4d\n",ncall));
#
# 3 (rows) x 2 (columns) matrix
  par(mfrow=c(3,2));
#
# Plot ODE dependent variables
  plot(tp,Sp,type="l",xlab="t (wk)",ylab="S(t)",
          lty=1,main="S(t)",lwd=2,col="black");
  plot(tp,Iap,type="l",xlab="t (wk)",ylab="Ia(t)",
          lty=1,main="Ia(t)",lwd=2,col="black");
  plot(tp,Isp,type="l",xlab="t (wk)",ylab="Is(t)",
          lty=1,main="Is(t)",lwd=2,col="black");
  plot(tp,Rp,type="l",xlab="t (wk)",ylab="R(t)",
          lty=1,main="R(t)",lwd=2,col="black");
  plot(tp,Dp,type="l",xlab="t (wk)",ylab="D(t)",
          lty=1,main="D(t)",lwd=2,col="black");
  plot(tp,Sp+Iap+Isp+Rp+Dp,type="l",xlab="t (wk)",
```

```
                 ylab="sum",lty=1,main="sum",lwd=2,
                 col="black");
#
# ODE t derivatives
   Stp=rep(0,nout);
  Iatp=rep(0,nout);
  Istp=rep(0,nout);
   Rtp=rep(0,nout);
   Dtp=rep(0,nout);
  sump=rep(0,nout);
  for(it in 1:nout){
    Stp[it]=rp*Stot-rSIa*Sp[it]*Iap[it]/Stot-
             rSIs*Sp[it]*Isp[it]/Stot+rR*Rp[it];
   Iatp[it]=rSIa*Sp[it]*Iap[it]/Stot-
             rIsIa*Iap[it]-rRIa*Iap[it]-
             rDIa*Iap[it];
   Istp[it]=rSIs*Sp[it]*Isp[it]/Stot+
             rIsIa*Iap[it]-rRIs*Isp[it]-
             rDIs*Isp[it];
    Rtp[it]=rRIa*Iap[it]+rRIs*Isp[it]-
             rR*Rp[it];
    Dtp[it]=rDIa*Iap[it]+rDIs*Isp[it];
   sump[it]=Stp[it]+Iatp[it]+Istp[it]+
             Rtp[it]+Dtp[it];
  }
#
# Plot ODE t derivatives
  plot(tp,Stp,type="l",xlab="t (wk)",
       ylab="dS(t)/dt",lty=1,main="dS(t)/dt",
       lwd=2,col="black");
  plot(tp,Iatp,type="l",xlab="t (wk)",
       ylab="dIa(t)/dt",lty=1,main="dIa(t)/dt",
       lwd=2,col="black");
  plot(tp,Istp,type="l",xlab="t (wk)",
```

```
          ylab="dIs(t)/dt",lty=1,main="dIs(t)/dt",
          lwd=2,col="black");
   plot(tp,Rtp,type="l",xlab="t (wk)",
          ylab="dR(t)/dt",lty=1,main="dR(t)/dt",
          lwd=2,col="black");
   plot(tp,Dtp,type="l",xlab="t (wk)",
          ylab="dD(t)/dt",lty=1,main="dD(t)/dt",
          lwd=2,col="black");
   plot(tp,sump,type="l",xlab="t (wk)",
          ylab="dsum(t)/dt",lty=1,main="dsum(t)/dt",
          lwd=2,col="black",ylim=Stot*c(-0.01,0.01));
```

Listing 2.1: Main program for eqs. (1.1), (1.2) with derivative calculation

The extended code of Listing 2.1 has the following calculation and display of t derivatives at the end.

- Computation and display of the t derivatives of eqs. (1.1) is added after the plotting of Listing 1.1, starting with arrays for the derivatives.

```
#
# ODE t derivatives
   Stp=rep(0,nout);
   Iatp=rep(0,nout);
   Istp=rep(0,nout);
   Rtp=rep(0,nout);
   Dtp=rep(0,nout);
   sump=rep(0,nout);
```

The previous designation of the plotting matrix, par(mfrow=c(3,2)); in Listing 1.1, remains in effect.
- The calculation of the derivatives is taken from ode1a of Listing 1.2.

```
for(it in 1:nout){
  Stp[it]=rp*Stot-rSIa*Sp[it]*Iap[it]/Stot-
          rSIs*Sp[it]*Isp[it]/Stot+rR*Rp[it];
  Iatp[it]=rSIa*Sp[it]*Iap[it]/Stot-
          rIsIa*Iap[it]-rRIa*Iap[it]-
          rDIa*Iap[it];
  Istp[it]=rSIs*Sp[it]*Isp[it]/Stot+
          rIsIa*Iap[it]-rRIs*Isp[it]-
          rDIs*Isp[it];
  Rtp[it]=rRIa*Iap[it]+rRIs*Isp[it]-
          rR*Rp[it];
  Dtp[it]=rDIa*Iap[it]+rDIs*Isp[it];
  sump[it]=Stp[it]+Iatp[it]+Istp[it]+
          Rtp[it]+Dtp[it];
}
```

For example, the code for $\dfrac{dS(t)}{dt}$ from ode1a

```
St=rp-rSIa*S*Ia-rSIs*S*Is+rR*R;
```

is programmed as

```
Stp[it]=rp*Stot-rSIa*Sp[it]*Iap[it]/Stot-
        rSIs*Sp[it]*Isp[it]/Stot+rR*Rp[it];
```

A subscript for t, p[it], is added to the LHS derivative and each RHS ODE dependent variable. Stot is used so that the derivative $\dfrac{dS(t)}{dt}$ includes a multiplication by Stot (through the RHS). That is, integration of this derivative gives $S(t)$ scaled by Stot. Also, the sum of the derivatives is programmed as sump[it].

- The t derivative vectors are plotted.

```
#
# Plot ODE t derivatives
  plot(tp,Stp,type="l",xlab="t (wk)",
```

```
        ylab="dS(t)/dt",lty=1,main="dS(t)/dt",
        lwd=2,col="black");
  plot(tp,Iatp,type="l",xlab="t (wk)",
        ylab="dIa(t)/dt",lty=1,main="dIa(t)/dt",
        lwd=2,col="black");
  plot(tp,Istp,type="l",xlab="t (wk)",
        ylab="dIs(t)/dt",lty=1,main="dIs(t)/dt",
        lwd=2,col="black");
  plot(tp,Rtp,type="l",xlab="t (wk)",
        ylab="dR(t)/dt",lty=1,main="dR(t)/dt",
        lwd=2,col="black");
  plot(tp,Dtp,type="l",xlab="t (wk)",
        ylab="dD(t)/dt",lty=1,main="dD(t)/dt",
        lwd=2,col="black");
  plot(tp,sump,type="l",xlab="t (wk)",
        ylab="dsum(t)/dt",lty=1,main="dsum(t)/dt",
        lwd=2,col="black",ylim=Stot*c(-0.01,0.01));
```

For example, $\dfrac{dS(t)}{dt}$ is plotted against t with

```
  plot(tp,Stp,type="l",xlab="t (wk)",
        ylab="dS(t)/dt",lty=1,main="dS(t)/dt",
        lwd=2,col="black");
```

The vertical scale of sump is defined by ylim=Stot*c(-0.01,0.01)) so that Stot*rp is plotted (see Appendix A1).

This completes the discussion of the additional code in Listing 2.1 for the calculation and plotting of the t derivatives $\dfrac{dS(t)}{dt}$, $\dfrac{dI_a(t)}{dt}$, $\dfrac{dI_s(t)}{dt}$, $\dfrac{dR(t)}{dt}$, $\dfrac{dD(t)}{dt}$.

(2.1.2) ODE routine

The ODE routine `ode1a` in Listing 1.2 is called by `lsodes` in the main program of Listing 2.1.

The output from the main program of Listing 2.1 and ODE routine `ode1a` of Listing 1.2 is considered next.

(2.1.3) Numerical, graphical output

The numerical output for $S(t)$, $I_a(t)$, $I_s(t)$, $R(t)$, $D(t)$ is the same as in Table 1.6 and is not repeated here. The graphical ouput for $S(t)$, $I_a(t)$, $I_s(t)$, $R(t)$, $D(t)$ is the same as in Fig. 1.1 and is not repeated here. The graphical output for the t derivatives $\dfrac{dS(t)}{dt}$, $\dfrac{dI_a(t)}{dt}$, $\dfrac{dI_s(t)}{dt}$, $\dfrac{dR(t)}{dt}$, $\dfrac{dD(t)}{dt}$ is in Fig. 2.1-1.

The derivatives $\dfrac{dS(t)}{dt}$, $\dfrac{dI_a(t)}{dt}$, $\dfrac{dIs(t)}{dt}$, $\dfrac{dR(t)}{dt}$, $\dfrac{dN(t)}{dt}$, approach a steady state (that could be further confirmed by extending the interval in t beyond `tf=52` set in Listing 2.1 (left as an exercise).

Figs. 1.1 and 2.1 indicate a maximum (peak) in the dependent variables $I_a(t)$, $I_s(t)$, and the corresponding derivatives $\dfrac{dI_a(t)}{dt}$, $\dfrac{dIs(t)}{dt}$, at approximatly 25 wks. The source of these maxima is considered next by studying the RHS terms of eqs. (1.1).

For the change to `rSIa=rSIs=0.5`, the output for $S(t)$, $I_a(t)$, $I_s(t)$, $R(t)$, $D(t)$ is the same as Table 1.7 and Fig. 1.2 and is not repeated here. The graphical output for $dS(t)/dt$, $dI_a(t)/dt$, $dI_s(t)/dt$, $dR(t)/dt$, $dD(t)/dt$ is in Fig 2.1-2.

The reduction in the derivatives $dS(t)/dt$, $dI_a(t)/dt$, $dI_s(t)/dt$, $dR(t)/dt$, $dD(t)/dt$ is clear (compare Figs. 2.1-1, 2.1-2).

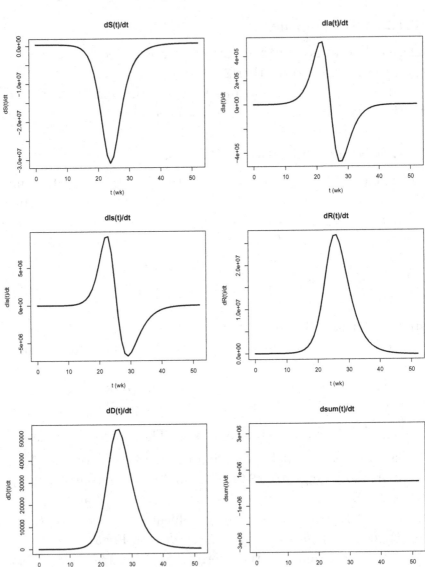

Figure   2.1-1: $dS(t)/dt, dI_a(t)/dt, dI_s(t)/dt, dR(t)/dt, dD(t)/dt$ from eqs. (1.1)

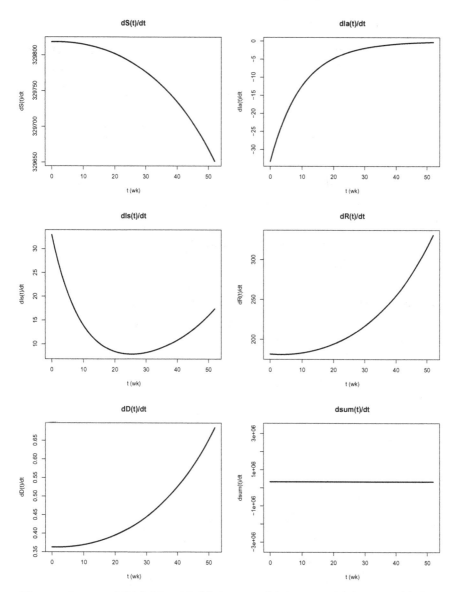

Figure 2.1-2: $dS(t)/dt$, $dI_a(t)/dt$, $dI_s(t)/dt$, $dR(t)/dt$, $dD(t)/dt$, rSIa=rSIs=0.5 from eqs. (1.1)

(2.1.4) Analysis of ODE LHS, RHS terms

The LHS t derivatives plotted in Fig. 2.1 have properties determined by the RHS terms of eqs. (1.1). These terms are computed and plotted by the following addition to the main program of Listing 2.1.

```
#
# ODE LHS, RHS terms
  par(mfrow=c(1,1));
#
# dS(t)/dt
  St_tm=matrix(0,nrow=nout,ncol=4);
  for(it in 1:nout){
    St_tm[it,1]=rp*Stot;
    St_tm[it,2]=-rSIa*Sp[it]*Iap[it]/Stot;
    St_tm[it,3]=-rSIs*Sp[it]*Isp[it]/Stot;
    St_tm[it,4]=+rR*Rp[it];
  }
   matplot(tp,St_tm,xlab="t (wk)",
           ylab="dS(t)/dt terms",
           col="black");
  matpoints(tp,St_tm,type="l",lty=1,
            lwd=2,col="black");
  legend('topright',legend=
         c('1 - rp',
           '2 - -rSIa*Sp[it]*Iap[it]',
           '3 - -rSIs*Sp[it]*Isp[it]',
           '4 - +rR*Rp[it]'));
#
# dIa(t)/dt
  Iat_tm=matrix(0,nrow=nout,ncol=4);
  for(it in 1:nout){
    Iat_tm[it,1]=rSIa*Sp[it]*Iap[it]/Stot;
    Iat_tm[it,2]=-rIsIa*Iap[it];
```

```
  Iat_tm[it,3]=-rRIa*Iap[it];
  Iat_tm[it,4]=-rDIa*Iap[it];
}
matplot(tp,Iat_tm,xlab="t (wk)",
        ylab="dIa(t)/dt terms",
        col="black");
matpoints(tp,Iat_tm,type="l",lty=1,
          lwd=2,col="black");
legend('topright',legend=
     c('1 - rSIa*Sp[it]*Iap[it]',
       '2 - -rIsIa*Iap[it]',
       '3 - -rRIa*Iap[it]',
       '4 - -rDIa*Iap[it]'));
```
```
#
# dIs(t)/dt
  Ist_tm=matrix(0,nrow=nout,ncol=4);
  for(it in 1:nout){
    Ist_tm[it,1]=rSIs*Sp[it]*Isp[it]/Stot;
    Ist_tm[it,2]=+rIsIa*Iap[it];
    Ist_tm[it,3]=-rRIs*Isp[it];
    Ist_tm[it,4]=-rDIs*Isp[it];
  }
  matplot(tp,Ist_tm,xlab="t (wk)",
          ylab="dIs(t)/dt terms",
          col="black");
  matpoints(tp,Ist_tm,type="l",lty=1,
            lwd=2,col="black");
  legend('topright',legend=
       c('1 - rSIs*Sp[it]*Isp[it]',
         '2 - +rIsIa*Iap[it]',
         '3 - -rRIs*Isp[it]',
         '4 - -rDIs*Isp[it]'));
#
# dR(t)/dt
```

```
Rt_tm=matrix(0,nrow=nout,ncol=3);
for(it in 1:nout){
  Rt_tm[it,1]=rRIa*Iap[it];
  Rt_tm[it,2]=rRIs*Isp[it];
  Rt_tm[it,3]=-rR*Rp[it];
}
matplot(tp,Rt_tm,xlab="t (wk)",
        ylab="dR(t)/dt terms",
        col="black");
matpoints(tp,Rt_tm,type="l",lty=1,
          lwd=2,col="black");
legend('topright',legend=
       c('1 - rRIa*Iap[it]',
         '2 - rRIs*Isp[it]',
         '3 - -rR*Rp[it]'));
#
# dD(t)/dt
  Dt_tm=matrix(0,nrow=nout,ncol=2);
  for(it in 1:nout){
    Dt_tm[it,1]=rDIa*Iap[it];
    Dt_tm[it,2]=rDIs*Isp[it];
  }
  matplot(tp,Dt_tm,xlab="t (wk)",
          ylab="dD(t)/dt terms",
          col="black");
  matpoints(tp,Dt_tm,type="l",lty=1,
            lwd=2,col="black");
  legend('topright',legend=
         c('1 - rDIa*Iap[it]',
           '2 - rDIs*Isp[it]'));
```

Listing 2.2: Extension of main program with calculation of ODE RHS terms

We can note the following details for this extension to the main program of Listing 2.1.

- The format is a 1×1 plot matrix on a page. The four RHS terms of eq. (1.1-1) are then computed and placed in array St_tm (tm denotes a RHS term). The terms are taken from the programming of eq. (1.1-1) near the end of Listing 2.1.

```
Stp[it]=rp*Stot-rSIa*Sp[it]*Iap[it]/Stot-
        rSIs*Sp[it]*Isp[it]/Stot+rR*Rp[it];

#
# ODE LHS, RHS terms
  par(mfrow=c(1,1));
#
# dS(t)/dt
  St_tm=matrix(0,nrow=nout,ncol=4);
  for(it in 1:nout){
    St_tm[it,1]=rp*Stot;
    St_tm[it,2]=-rSIa*Sp[it]*Iap[it]/Stot;
    St_tm[it,3]=-rSIs*Sp[it]*Isp[it]/Stot;
    St_tm[it,4]=+rR*Rp[it];
  }
```

The sum of the four RHS terms of eq. (1.1-1) is not included in the plotting since it complicates the plot (the sum equals the left t derivative $\dfrac{dS(t)}{dt}$ which is already plotted in Fig. 2.1-1).

- Matrix St_tm is plotted parametrically against time, tp.

```
matplot(tp,St_tm,xlab="t (wk)",
        ylab="dS(t)/dt terms",
        col="black");
matpoints(tp,St_tm,type="l",lty=1,
          lwd=2,col="black");
```

```
legend('topright',legend=
   c('1 - rp',
     '2 - -rSIa*Sp[it]*Iap[it]',
     '3 - -rSIs*Sp[it]*Isp[it]',
     '4 - +rR*Rp[it]'));
```

`matplot` provides discrete points with numbers. `matpoints` provides lines connecting the points from `matplot` through the arguments `type="l",lty=1,` `lwd=2,` The legend identifies the four RHS terms (`Stot` is not included in the legend).

The graphical output is in Fig. 2.2-1.
We can note the following details about this figure.

- The largest contributor identified with 3 is

    `St_tm[it,3]=-rSIs*Sp[it]*Isp[it]/Stot;`

or

$$-r_{SI_s}SI_s$$

in eq. (1.1-1).
- The second largest contributor identified with 2 is

    `St_tm[it,2]=-rSIa*Sp[it]*Iap[it]/Stot;`

or

$$-r_{SI_a}SI_a$$

in eq. (1.1-1).
- The first and fourth terms, identified with 1,4, remain at essentially zero.

    `St_tm[it,1]=Stot*rp;`

    `St_tm[it,4]=+rR*Rp[it];`

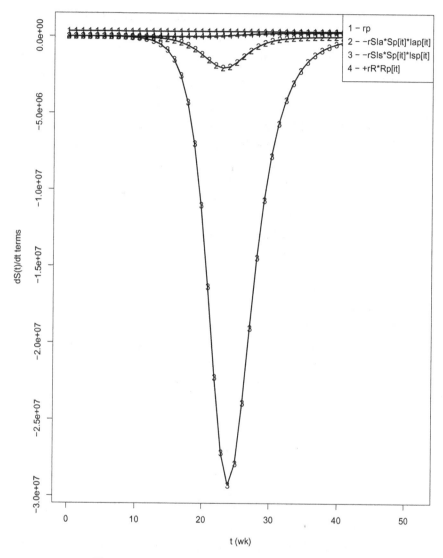

Figure 2.2-1: RHS terms of eq. (1.1-1)

or

$$r_p$$

$$+r_R R$$

in eq. (1.1-1).

In summary, the relative contributions of the four RHS terms of eq. (1.1-1) can be readily ascertained from the composite plot of Fig. 2.2-1. This comparison of terms facilitates the formulation, and possibly the revision, of eq. (1.1-1).

A similar analysis of eq. (1.1-2) follows.

- The four RHS terms of eq. (1.1-2) are computed and placed in array Iat_tm. The terms are taken from the programming of eq. (1.1-2) near the end of Listing 2.1.

```
Iatp[it]=rSIa*Sp[it]*Iap[it]/Stot-
         rIsIa*Iap[it]-rRIa*Iap[it]-
         rDIa*Iap[it];
```

```
#
# dIa(t)/dt
  Iat_tm=matrix(0,nrow=nout,ncol=4);
  for(it in 1:nout){
    Iat_tm[it,1]=rSIa*Sp[it]*Iap[it]/Stot;
    Iat_tm[it,2]=-rIsIa*Iap[it];
    Iat_tm[it,3]=-rRIa*Iap[it];
    Iat_tm[it,4]=-rDIa*Iap[it];
  }
```

The sum of the four RHS terms of eq. (1.1-2) is not included in the plotting since it complicates the plot (the sum equals the left t derivative $\dfrac{dI_a(t)}{dt}$ which is already plotted in Fig. 2.1-1).

- Matrix Iat_tm is plotted parametrically against time, tp.

```
matplot(tp,Iat_tm,xlab="t (wk)",
        ylab="dIa(t)/dt terms",
        col="black");
matpoints(tp,Iat_tm,type="l",lty=1,
          lwd=2,col="black");
legend('topright',legend=
```

```
c('1 - rSIa*Sp[it]*Iap[it]',
  '2 - -rIsIa*Iap[it]',
  '3 - -rRIa*Iap[it]',
  '4 - -rDIa*Iap[it]'));
```

The legend identifies the four RHS terms (`Stot` is not included in the legend).

The graphical output is in Fig. 2.2-2.

We can note the following details about this figure.

- The largest contributor identified with 1 is

    ```
    Iat_tm[it,1]=rSIa*Sp[it]*Iap[it]/Stot;
    ```

  or

  $$r_{SI_a} SI_a$$

  in eq. (1.1-2). This term is positive reflecting the conversion of susceptibles to asymptomatic infecteds.
- The second and third terms identified with 2,3 are negative reflecting the conversion of asymptomatic infecteds to symptomatic infecteds and recovereds.

    ```
    Iat_tm[it,2]=-rIsIa*Iap[it];
    Iat_tm[it,3]=-rRIa*Iap[it];
    ```

  or

  $$-r_{I_s I_a} I_a - r_{RI_a} I_a$$

  in eq. (1.1-2).

In summary, the relative contributions of the four RHS terms of eq. (1.1-2) can be readily ascertained from the composite plot of Fig. 2.2-2. This comparison of terms facilitates the formulation, and possibly the revision, of eq. (1.1-2).

A similar analysis of eq. (1.1-3) follows.

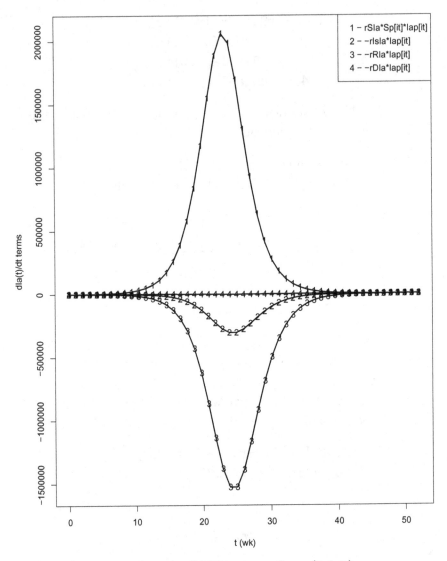

Figure 2.2-2: RHS terms of eq. (1.1-2)

- The four RHS terms of eq. (1.1-3) are computed and placed in array Ist_tm. The terms are taken from the programming of eq. (1.1-3) near the end of Listing 2.1.

```
Istp[it]=rSIs*Sp[it]*Isp[it]/Stot+
```

```
    rIsIa*Iap[it]-rRIs*Isp[it]-
    rDIs*Isp[it];

#
# dIs(t)/dt
  Ist_tm=matrix(0,nrow=nout,ncol=4);
  for(it in 1:nout){
    Ist_tm[it,1]=rSIs*Sp[it]*Isp[it]/Stot;
    Ist_tm[it,2]=+rIsIa*Iap[it];
    Ist_tm[it,3]=-rRIs*Isp[it];
    Ist_tm[it,4]=-rDIs*Isp[it];
  }
```

The sum of the four RHS terms of eq. (1.1-3) is not included in the plotting since it complicates the plot (the sum equals the left t derivative $\dfrac{dI_s(t)}{dt}$ which is already plotted in Fig. 2.1-1).

• Matrix Ist_tm is plotted parametrically against time, tp.

```
  matplot(tp,Ist_tm,xlab="t (wk)",
          ylab="dIs(t)/dt terms",
          col="black");
  matpoints(tp,Ist_tm,type="l",lty=1,
            lwd=2,col="black");
  legend('topright',legend=
      c('1 - rSIs*Sp[it]*Isp[it]',
        '2 - +rIsIa*Iap[it]',
        '3 - -rRIs*Isp[it]',
        '4 - -rDIs*Isp[it]'));
```

The legend identifies the four RHS terms (Stot is not included in the legend).

The graphical output is in Fig. 2.2-3.
We can note the following details about this figure.

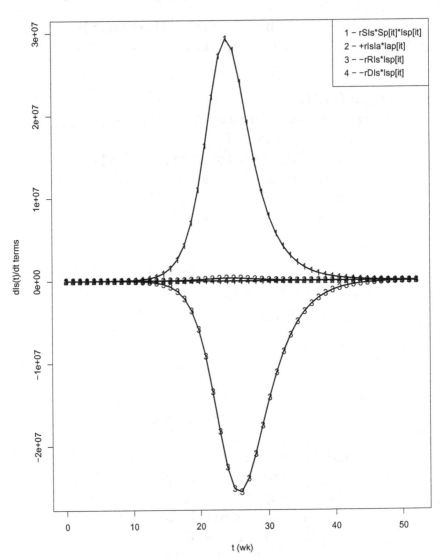

Figure 2.2-3: RHS terms of eq. (1.1-3)

- The largest contributor with 1 is

    ```
    Ist_tm[it,1]=rSIs*Sp[it]*Isp[it]/Stot;
    ```

  or

$$r_{SI_s}SI_s$$

in eq. (1.1-3). This term is positive reflecting the conversion of susceptibles to symptomatic infecteds.

- The third term identified with 3 is negative reflecting the conversion of symptomatic infecteds to recovereds.

```
Ist_tm[it,3]=-rRIs*Isp[it];
```

or

$$-r_{RI_s} I_s$$

in eq. (1.1-3).

In summary, the relative contributions of the four RHS terms of eq. (1.1-3) can be readily ascertained from the composite plot of Fig. 2.2-3. This comparison of terms facilitates the formulation, and possibly the revision, of eq. (1.1-3).

An analysis of eq. (1.1-4) follows.

- The three RHS terms of eq. (1.1-4) are computed and placed in array R_tm. The terms are taken from the programming of eq. (1.1-4) near the end of Listing 2.1.

```
Rtp[it]=rRIa*Iap[it]+rRIs*Isp[it]-
        rR*Rp[it];
```

```
#
# dR(t)/dt
  Rt_tm=matrix(0,nrow=nout,ncol=3);
  for(it in 1:nout){
    Rt_tm[it,1]=rRIa*Iap[it];
    Rt_tm[it,2]=rRIs*Isp[it];
    Rt_tm[it,3]=-rR*Rp[it];
  }
```

The sum of the three RHS terms of eq. (1.1-4) is not included in the plotting since it complicates the plot (the sum equals the left t derivative $\dfrac{dR(t)}{dt}$ which is already plotted in Fig. 2.1-1).

- Matrix Rt_tm is plotted parametrically against time, tp.

```
matplot(tp,Rt_tm,xlab="t (wk)",
        ylab="dR(t)/dt terms",
        col="black");
matpoints(tp,Rt_tm,type="l",lty=1,
          lwd=2,col="black");
legend('topright',legend=
    c('1 - rRIa*Iap[it]',
      '2 - rRIs*Isp[it]',
      '3 - -rR*Rp[it]'));
```

The legend identifies the three RHS terms (Stot is not included in the legend).

The graphical output is in Fig. 2.2-4.
We can note the following details about this figure.

- The largest contributor to the sum of terms identified with 2 is

      Rt_tm[it,2]=rRIs*Isp[it];

or

$$r_{RI_s}I_s$$

in eq. (1.1-4).
- The second largest contributor to the sum of terms identified with 1 is

      Rt_tm[it,1]=rRIa*Iap[it];

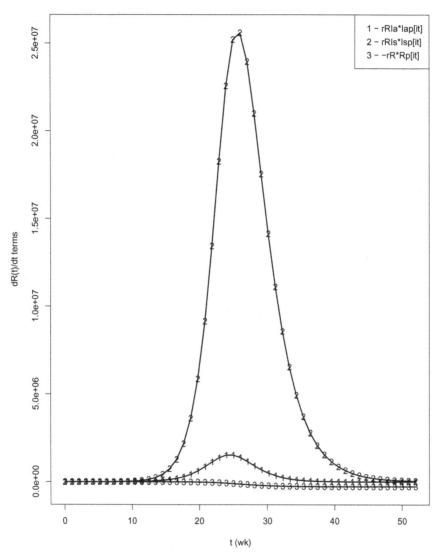

Figure 2.2-4: RHS terms of eq. (1.1-4)

or

$$r_{RI_a} I_a$$

in eq. (1.1-4).

- The third term, identified with 3, remains at essentially zero.

      ```
      Rt_tm[it,3]=-rR*Rp[it];
      ```

  or

  $$-r_R R$$

  in eq. (1.1-4).

In summary, the relative contributions of the three RHS terms of eq. (1.1-4) can be readily ascertained from the composite plot of Fig. 2.2-4. This comparison of terms facilitates the formulation, and possibly the revision, of eq. (1.1-4).

An analysis of eq. (1.1-5) follows.

- The two RHS terms of eq. (1.1-5) are computed and placed in array Dt_tm. The terms are taken from the programming of eq. (1.1-5) near the end of Listing 2.1.

      ```
      Dtp[it]=rDIa*Iap[it]+rDIs*Isp[it];
      ```

  ```
  #
  # dD(t)/dt
    Dt_tm=matrix(0,nrow=nout,ncol=2);
    for(it in 1:nout){
      Dt_tm[it,1]=rDIa*Iap[it];
      Dt_tm[it,2]=rDIs*Isp[it];
    }
  ```

  The sum of the two RHS terms of eq. (1.1-5) is not included in the plotting since it complicates the plot (the sum equals the left t derivative $\dfrac{dD(t)}{dt}$ which is already plotted in Fig. 2.1-1).

- Matrix Dt_tm is plotted parametrically against time, tp.

      ```
      matplot(tp,Dt_tm,xlab="t (wk)",
              ylab="dD(t)/dt terms",
      ```

```
        col="black");
matpoints(tp,Dt_tm,type="l",lty=1,
        lwd=2,col="black");
legend('topright',legend=
    c('1 - rDIa*Iap[it]',
      '2 - rDIs*Isp[it]'));
```

The legend identifies the two RHS terms (Stot is not included in the legend).

The graphical output is in Fig. 2.2-5.
We can note the following details about this figure.

- The larger contributor identified with 2 is

    Dt_tm[it,2]=rDIs*Isp[it];

  or

  $$r_{DI_s} I_s$$

  in eq. (1.1-5).
- The smaller contributor identified with 1 is

    Dt_tm[it,1]=rDIa*Iap[it];

  or

  $$r_{DI_a} I_a$$

  in eq. (1.1-5).

In summary, the relative contributions of the two RHS terms of eq. (1.1-5) can be readily ascertained from the composite plot of Fig. 2.2-5. This comparison of terms facilitates the formulation, and possibly the revision, of eq. (1.1-5).

This completes the analysis of the RHS terms and LHS derivatives of eqs. (1.1), with the objective of explaining the origin of the properties of $S(t)$, $Ia(t)$, $Is(t)$, $R(t)$, $D(t)$.

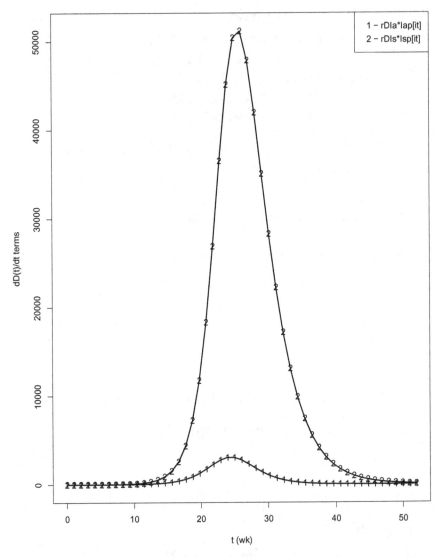

Figure 2.2-5: RHS terms of eq. (1.1-5)

(2.2) Summary and Conclusions

A methodology for elucidating the RHS terms and LHS derivatives of the basic ODE model, eqs. (1.1), (1.2), is presented. The analysis of these terms indicates which terms are most important in determining the time evolution of the solutions $S(t)$, $Ia(t)$, $Is(t)$, $R(t)$, $D(t)$. Of particular interest are (1) the signs of the derivatives which determine whether the variables decrease ($S(t)$ with negative feedback) or increase ($Ia(t)$, $Is(t)$, $R(t)$, $D(t)$ with positive feedback) with t, and (2) the magnitudes of the derivatives which determine the time scale of the solutions ($0 \leq t \leq 52$ wks).

Chapter 3

Variants of the Basic ODE Model

(3) Introduction

The ODE model, eqs. (1.1), (1.2), implemented in the R routines of Chapters 1, 2, can be used for studies of (1) parameter variations and (2) structural changes. For (1), the example of the susceptibles to asymptomatic and symptomatic rate constants changes, `rSIa= rSIs =1` to `rSIa= rSIs=0.5` in Chapter 1, demonstrates a large reduction in recovereds and deaths (Tables 1.6, 1.7 and Figs. 1.1, 1.2).

These cases are based on the assumption that all susceptibles can become infecteds. Consideration is first given to the case when a fraction of the susceptibles do not become infected.

(3.1) Limited susceptibles infection

The rate of conversion of susceptible to infecteds is determined by the terms in Table 3.1 which are not limited to a range of values for $S(t)$, $I_a(t)$ or $I_s(t)$. Consideration is now given to rates that are limited in $S(t)$.

$$-r_{SI_a} S I_a \quad \text{eq. (1.1-1)}$$

$$-r_{SI_s} S I_s \quad \text{eq. (1.1-1)}$$

$$+r_{SI_a} S I_a \quad \text{eq. (1.1-2)}$$

$$+r_{SI_s} S I_s \quad \text{eq. (1.1-3)}$$

Table 3.1: Susceptible to infected transmission rates

Eqs. (1.1) modified with logistic rates are stated as eqs. (3.1).

$$\frac{dS}{dt} = r_p - r_{SI_a}(S - S_{lim})I_a - r_{SI_s}(S - S_{lim})I_s + r_R R \quad (3.1\text{-}1)$$

$$\frac{dI_a}{dt} = r_{SI_a}(S - S_{lim})I_a - r_{I_s I_a}I_a - r_{DI_a}I_a \quad (3.1\text{-}2)$$

$$\frac{dI_s}{dt} = r_{SI_s}(S - S_{lim})I_s + r_{I_s I_a}I_a - r_{DI_s}I_s \quad (3.1\text{-}3)$$

$$\frac{dR}{dt} = r_{RI_a}I_a + r_{RI_s}I_s - r_R R \quad (3.1\text{-}4)$$

$$\frac{dD}{dt} = r_{DI_a}I_a + r_{DI_s}I_s \quad (3.1\text{-}5)$$

For example, the logistic rate $-r_{SI_a}(S - S_{lim})I_a$ in eq. (1.1-1) includes the threshold S_{lim} so that the rate decreases as $S(t) \to S_{lim}$. The effect of the limited rate on $S(t)$, $I_a(t)$ or $I_s(t)$ can be observed with the following changes in the main program of Listing 1.1 and ODE routine of Listing 1.2.

(3.1.1) Main program

Two changes in the main program of Listing 1.1 for the addition of S_{lim} are indicated next.

- The parameter list is modified to include S_{lim}.

```
#
# Model parameters
#
# S(t)
   rp=0.001;
   rSIa=1;
   rSIs=1;
   rR=0.001;
   Stot=3.3e+08;
   ncase=1;
   if(ncase==1){
     Slim=0;}
   if(ncase==2){
     Slim=0.5;}
#
# Ia(t)
#
# Is(t)
   rIsIa=0.1;
#
# R(t)
   rRIa=0.5;
   rRIs=0.5;
#
# D(t)
   rDIa=0.001;
   rDIs=0.001;
```

Listing 3.1: Parameters in the main program for eqs. (1.1), (1.2)

For `ncase=1`, `SLIM=0`; is a repeat of the base case of Listing 1.1. The output is in Table 1.6 and Fig. 1.1. For `ncase=2`, `Slim=0.5` limits the susceptibles to infecteds rate, which could model, for example, the effect of enforced separation that reduces the rate of interaction of susceptibles with infecteds ("social distancing"). The numerical and graphical output for this case is considered subsequently.

- Since `Slim=0.5` slows the dynamics of the modeled system, the time scale is extended from $t_f = 52$ wks to $t_f = 4(52) = 208$ wks.

```
#
# Temporal grid
  if(ncase==1){
    nout=51;t0=0;tf=52;}
  if(ncase==2){
    nout=51;t0=0;tf=4*52;}
  tout=seq(from=t0,to=tf,by=(tf-t0)/(nout-1));
```

(3.1.2) ODE routine

The ODE routine, `ode1a`, called by `lsodes` in Listing 3.1, is listed next.

```
  ode1a=function(t,y,parm) {
#
# Function ode1a computes the t derivative
# vectors of S(t),Ia(t),Is(t),R(t),D(t)
#
# One vector to five scalars
  S=y[1];
  Ia=y[2];
```

```
    Is=y[3];
     R=y[4];
     D=y[5];
#
# ODEs
   St=rp-rSIa*(S-Slim)*Ia-
          rSIs*(S-Slim)*Is+rR*R;
   Iat=rSIa*(S-Slim)*Ia-rIsIa*Ia-
       rRIa*Ia-rDIa*Ia;
   Ist=rSIs*(S-Slim)*Is+rIsIa*Ia-
       rRIs*Is-rDIs*Is;
    Rt=rRIa*Ia+rRIs*Is-rR*R;
    Dt=rDIa*Ia+rDIs*Is;
#
# Five scalars to one vector
   yt=rep(0,5);
   yt[1]=St;
   yt[2]=Iat;
   yt[3]=Ist
   yt[4]=Rt;
   yt[5]=Dt;
#
# Increment calls to ncall
   ncall <<- ncall+1;
#
# Return ODE t vector
   return(list(c(yt)));
#
# End of ode1a
   }
```

Listing 3.2: ODE routine ode1a for eqs. (3.1)

ode1a of Listing 1.2 is extended to include the logistic rate with S_{lim} in eqs. (3.1).

```
#
# ODEs
   St=rp-rSIa*(S-Slim)*Ia-
        rSIs*(S-Slim)*Is+rR*R;
  Iat=rSIa*(S-Slim)*Ia-rIsIa*Ia-
      rRIa*Ia-rDIa*Ia;
  Ist=rSIs*(S-Slim)*Is+rIsIa*Ia-
      rRIs*Is-rDIs*Is;
   Rt=rRIa*Ia+rRIs*Is-rR*R;
   Dt=rDIa*Ia+rDIs*Is;
```

The numerical and graphical ouput for ncase=2 follows.

(3.1.3) Numerical, graphical output

[1] 51

[1] 6

t		
0.0		
S(t)	Ia(t)	Is(t)
R(t)	D(t)	sum
3.30e+08	3.30e+02	3.30e+01
0.00e+00	0.00e+00	3.30e+08

t		
41.6		
S(t)	Ia(t)	Is(t)
R(t)	D(t)	sum
3.44e+08	1.56e+01	8.64e+02
1.07e+04	2.17e+01	3.44e+08

```
            t
          83.2
         S(t)          Ia(t)          Is(t)
         R(t)           D(t)           sum
      3.57e+08       3.10e+00       1.14e+04
      8.49e+04       1.73e+02       3.57e+08


            t
         124.8
         S(t)          Ia(t)          Is(t)
         R(t)           D(t)           sum
      3.67e+08       3.03e+00       7.30e+05
      3.37e+06       6.81e+03       3.71e+08


            t
         166.4
         S(t)          Ia(t)          Is(t)
         R(t)           D(t)           sum
      3.06e+08       1.93e-01       2.94e+06
      7.58e+07       1.54e+05       3.85e+08


            t
         208.0
         S(t)          Ia(t)          Is(t)
         R(t)           D(t)           sum
      3.09e+08       1.15e-04       1.06e+05
      8.94e+07       1.89e+05       3.99e+08


ncall =   109
```

Table 3.1: Numerical output from Listings 3.1, 3.2, ncase=2

We can note the following details about this output.

- 51 t output points as the first dimension of the solution matrix out from lsodes as programmed in the main program of Listings 1.1, 3.1 (with nout=51).
- The solution matrix out returned by lsodes has 6 elements as a second dimension. The first element is the value of t. Elements 2 to 6 are $S(t), Ia(t), Is(t), R(t), D(t)$ from eqs. (3.1) (for each of the 51 output points).
- The solution is displayed for t=0,208*10/50=41.6,..., 208 as programmed in Listings 1.1, 3.1 (every tenth value of t is displayed as explained previously).
- ICs (1.2) are confirmed $(t = 0)$, as scaled by S_{tot}.
- $S(t), Ia(t), Is(t), R(t), D(t)$ sum to a near constant value in t, starting with $S(t = 0) = 3.3 \times 10^8$. This is an important test of eqs. (3.1) as discussed in the chapter Appendix A1.
- The deaths, $D(t)$, are about 1/500 of the recoverds, $R(t)$. For example, at $t = 208$, $D(t = 52)/R(t = 208) = 1.89 \times 10^5/8.94 \times 10^7 = 0.002114 \approx 1/500$.
- The computational effort as indicated by ncall = 109 is modest so that lsodes computed the solution to eqs. (3.1) efficiently.

The graphical output is in Fig. 3.1.

The solutions $S(t), Ia(t), Is(t), R(t), D(t)$ approach a steady state. The sum of the five dependent variables, sum, increases with t that is the result of the susceptible production term in eq. (3.1), r_p, as explained in Appendix A1.

In summary, the use of S_{lim} in eqs. (3.1) delays the response in t $(t_f = 52$ without S_{lim}, $t_f = 208$ with $S_{lim})$ and reduces the

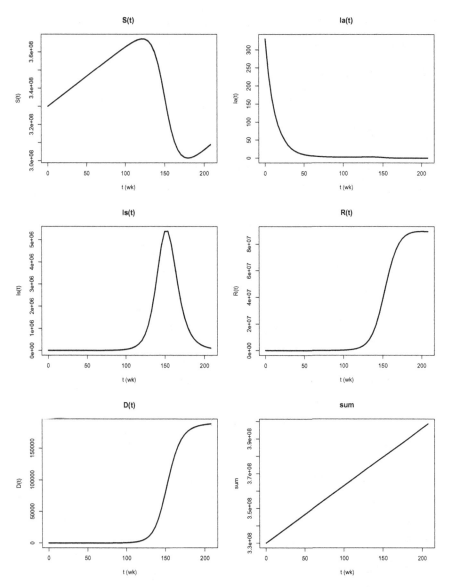

Figure 3.1: $S(t), Ia(t), Is(t), R(t), D(t)$ from eqs. (3.1)

final values of $R(t)$ and $S(t)$. For example, at the final values of t in Tables 1.6, 3.1,

```
Table 1.6, ncase=1
        t
      52.0
      S(t)           Ia(t)            Is(t)
      R(t)           D(t)              sum
  7.74e+07        2.93e+02        7.42e+04
  2.69e+08        5.52e+05        3.47e+08
```

```
Table 3.1, ncase=2
        t
      208.0
      S(t)           Ia(t)            Is(t)
      R(t)           D(t)              sum
  3.09e+08        1.15e-04        1.06e+05
  8.94e+07        1.89e+05        3.99e+08
```

The final deaths are reduced by `5.52e+05-1.89e+05=363000` or 65.8% of `5.52e+05`.

As a concluding case, S_{lim} is switched from 0.5 to 0 at $t = t_{swt} > 0$ representing the return of the logistic rates $(S - S_{lim})I_a$, $(S - S_{lim})I_s$ in eqs. (3.1-1,2,3) to the maximum values. This might represent, for example, the termination of the enforced separation ("social distancing"). The time of the switch, tswt, is designated in the following parameter list (for ncase=2 in Listing 3.1).

```
  ncase=2;
  if(ncase==1){
    Slim=0;}
  if(ncase==2){
    Slim=0.5;
    tswt=104;}
```

Listing 3.3: Addition of switch time tswt for ncase=2

In this case, the switch occurs at the mid point in t, tswt=104.
  The Slim switching is added to ode1a of Listing 3.2.

```
#
# ODEs
  if((ncase==2)&&(t>tswt)){Slim=0;}
  St=rp-rSIa*(S-Slim)*Ia-
        rSIs*(S-Slim)*Is+rR*R;
  Iat=rSIa*(S-Slim)*Ia-rIsIa*Ia-
      rRIa*Ia-rDIa*Ia;
  Ist=rSIs*(S-Slim)*Is+rIsIa*Ia-
      rRIs*Is-rDIs*Is;
  Rt=rRIa*Ia+rRIs*Is-rR*R;
  Dt=rDIa*Ia+rDIs*Is;
```

Listing 3.4: Addition of switch time tswt in ode1a

The numerical and graphical output with the changes in Listings
3.3, 3.4 follows.

[1] 51

[1] 6

	t	
	0.0	
S(t)	Ia(t)	Is(t)
R(t)	D(t)	sum
3.30e+08	3.30e+02	3.30e+01
0.00e+00	0.00e+00	3.30e+08

	t	
	41.6	
S(t)	Ia(t)	Is(t)
R(t)	D(t)	sum
3.44e+08	1.56e+01	8.64e+02
1.07e+04	2.17e+01	3.44e+08

```
          t
        83.2
        S(t)            Ia(t)            Is(t)
        R(t)            D(t)             sum
     3.57e+08        3.10e+00         1.14e+04
     8.49e+04        1.73e+02         3.57e+08


          t
        124.8
        S(t)            Ia(t)            Is(t)
        R(t)            D(t)             sum
     6.87e+07        7.97e+01         1.89e+07
     2.83e+08        5.70e+05         3.71e+08


          t
        166.4
        S(t)            Ia(t)            Is(t)
        R(t)            D(t)             sum
     8.30e+07        1.64e-04         8.76e+01
     3.01e+08        6.32e+05         3.85e+08


          t
        208.0
        S(t)            Ia(t)            Is(t)
        R(t)            D(t)             sum
     1.09e+08       -4.48e-07         3.59e-01
     2.89e+08        6.32e+05         3.99e+08


ncall =   235
```

Table 3.2: Numerical output from Listings 3.1 to 3.4, ncase=2

The graphical output is in Fig. 3.2.

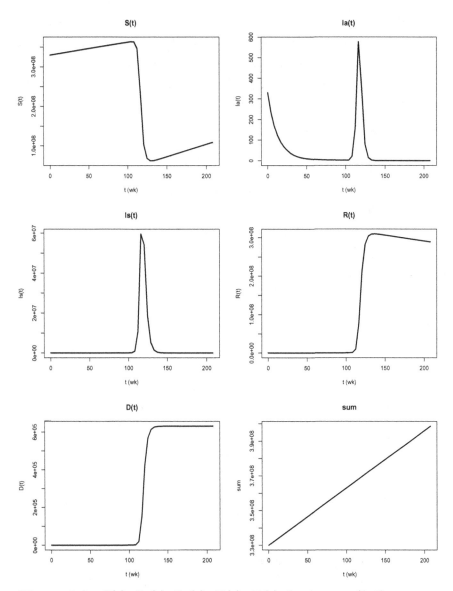

Figure 3.2: $S(t), Ia(t), Is(t), R(t), D(t)$ from eqs. (3.1), $t_{swt} = 104$

The sharp return near $t = 104$ to the $S_{lim} = 0$ solution of Table 1.6 can be observed in Fig. 3.2. In fact, the final recovereds and deaths are slightly higher because of the extended time scale ($t_f = 52$ extended to $t_f = 208$). Also, sum has a greater variation with the increased t as explained in Appendix A1.

Table 1.6, ncase=1

t		
52.0		
S(t)	Ia(t)	Is(t)
R(t)	D(t)	sum
7.74e+07	2.93e+02	7.42e+04
2.69e+08	5.52e+05	3.47e+08

Table 3.2, ncase=2, Tswt=104

t		
208.0		
S(t)	Ia(t)	Is(t)
R(t)	D(t)	sum
1.09e+08	-4.48e-07	3.59e-01
2.89e+08	6.32e+05	3.99e+08

For example, the deaths have a small increase, D(t=52)=5.52e+05, D(t=208)=6.32e+05.

In summary, t_{swt} is a sensitive parameter in determining the final solution, that is, the level at which the epidemic is contained.

(3.2) Summary and conclusions

The 5×5 ODE model of Chapter 1 is extended to include a limit on the rate of transition of susceptibles to infecteds as stated in eqs. (3.1) with S_{lim}. The time of application of this limit, t_{sw}, is also considered. The final (steady state) solutions are sensitive to both parameters (S_{lim}, t_{sw}).

Chapter 4

Postulated Vaccine/Therapeutic Drug Treatment

(4) Introduction

The model of eqs. (3.1) is extended to include a postulated vaccine/therapeutic drug treatment, which is implemented through a reduction of the rSIa, rSIs rate constants with t.

(4.1) ODE model with parameter time variation

The analysis of eqs. (3.1) indicates that the parameters rSIa, rSIs are important parameters in determing the course of the COVID-19 infection. We now consider a variation of these parameters with t which could represent, for example, the introduction of a vaccine or therapeutic drug treatment.

The time variation of the parameters rSIa, rSIs is implemented with the function

$$rate(t) = e^{-k_r(t-t_0)/(t_f-t_0)} \qquad (4.1)$$

k_r is defined as a parameter in the main program and $rate(t)$ is added to ode1a.

(4.1.1) Main program

The parameter set is defined in Listing 4.1.

```
#
# Model parameters
#
# S(t)
  rp=0.001;
  rSIa=1;
  rSIs=1;
  rR=0.001;
  Stot=3.3e+08;
  Slim=0;
  kr=2;
  ncase=1;
#
# Ia(t)
#
# Is(t)
  rIsIa=0.1;
#
# R(t)
  rRIa=0.5;
  rRIs=0.5;
#
# D(t)
  rDIa=0.001;
  rDIs=0.001;
```

Listing 4.1: Parameters for Listing 1.1

In particular, k_r is defined (and used in **ode1a**). The original time interval is retained, $0 \leq t \leq t_f = 52$.

(4.1.2) ODE routine

The ODE routine **ode1a** is an extension of the the routine of Listing 1.2.

```
ode1a=function(t,y,parm) {
#
# Function ode1a computes the t derivative
# vectors of S(t),Ia(t),Is(t),R(t),D(t)
#
# One vector to five scalars
  S=y[1];
  Ia=y[2];
  Is=y[3];
  R=y[4];
  D=y[5];
#
# ODEs
  if(ncase==1){rate=1;}
  if(ncase==2){rate=exp(-kr*(t-t0)/(tf-t0));}
  St=rp-rSIa*(S-Slim)*Ia*rate-
       rSIs*(S-Slim)*Is*rate+rR*R;
  Iat=rSIa*(S-Slim)*Ia*rate-rIsIa*Ia-
     rRIa*Ia-rDIa*Ia;
  Ist=rSIs*(S-Slim)*Is*rate+rIsIa*Ia-
     rRIs*Is-rDIs*Is;
  Rt=rRIa*Ia+rRIs*Is-rR*R;
  Dt=rDIa*Ia+rDIs*Is;
#
# Five scalars to one vector
  yt=rep(0,5);
  yt[1]=St;
  yt[2]=Iat;
```

```
  yt[3]=Ist
  yt[4]=Rt;
  yt[5]=Dt;
#
# Increment calls to ncall
  ncall <<- ncall+1;
#
# Return ODE t vector
  return(list(c(yt)));
#
# End of ode1a
  }
```

Listing 4.2: ODE routine **ode1a** including function (4.1)

Listing 4.2 is the same as Listing 1.2 except for the programming of the ODEs.

- Two cases are programmed. For **ncase=1** (defined in Listing 4.1), **rate=1** and this is a repeat of the base case of Listing 1.1.

```
#
# ODEs
  if(ncase==1){rate=1;}
  if(ncase==2){rate=exp(-kr*(t-t0)/(tf-t0));}
```

For **ncase=2**, eq. (4.1) is implemented. In particular, k_r is used and t is taken as the first argument of **ode1a**.

- Eq. (3.1-1) is programmed, with **rate** applied to the nonlinear **-rSIa*(S-Slim)*Ia** and **-rSIs*(S-Slim)*Is** logistic rates (**Slim=0**).

```
  St=rp-rSIa*(S-Slim)*Ia*rate-
       rSIs*(S-Slim)*Is*rate+rR*R;
```

- Eq. (3.1-2) is programmed, with **rate** applied to the non-linear `rSIa*(S-Slim)*Ia` logistic rate.

  ```
  Iat=rSIa*(S-Slim)*Ia*rate-rIsIa*Ia-
      rRIa*Ia-rDIa*Ia;
  ```

- Eq. (3.1-3) is programmed, with **rate** applied to the non-linear `rSIs*(S-Slim)*Is` logistic rate.

  ```
  Ist=rSIs*(S-Slim)*Is*rate+rIsIa*Ia-
      rRIs*Is-rDIs*Is;
  ```

- The programming of eqs. (3.1-4,5) remains unchanged.

The output from Listings 4.1, 4.2 follows.

(4.1.3) Numerical, graphical output

The output for **ncase=1** is the same as in Table 1.6, Fig. 1.1. The numerical output for **ncase=2** follows.

```
[1] 51

[1] 6
            t
          0.0
         S(t)          Ia(t)          Is(t)
         R(t)           D(t)           sum
     3.30e+08       3.30e+02       3.30e+01
     0.00e+00       0.00e+00       3.30e+08


            t
         10.4
         S(t)          Ia(t)          Is(t)
         R(t)           D(t)           sum
     3.33e+08       3.99e+03       1.09e+04
     2.82e+04       5.65e+01       3.33e+08
```

```
       t
      20.8
      S(t)           Ia(t)           Is(t)
      R(t)           D(t)            sum
   3.37e+08       2.66e+03        2.49e+04
   1.57e+05       3.15e+02        3.37e+08


       t
      31.2
      S(t)           Ia(t)           Is(t)
      R(t)           D(t)            sum
   3.40e+08       2.68e+02        7.37e+03
   2.47e+05       5.00e+02        3.40e+08


       t
      41.6
      S(t)           Ia(t)           Is(t)
      R(t)           D(t)            sum
   3.43e+08       1.21e+00        6.41e+02
   2.60e+05       5.32e+02        3.44e+08


       t
      52.0
      S(t)           Ia(t)           Is(t)
      R(t)           D(t)            sum
   3.47e+08       3.12e-02        3.45e+01
   2.58e+05       5.34e+02        3.47e+08


ncall =    84
```

Table 4.1: Numerical output from Listings 4.1, 4.2, ncase=2

We can note the following details about this output.

- 51 t output points as the first dimension of the solution matrix out from lsodes as programmed in the main program of Listings 1.1, 4.1 (with nout=51).
- The solution matrix out returned by lsodes has 6 elements as a second dimension. The first element is the value of t. Elements 2 to 6 are $S(t)$, $Ia(t)$, $Is(t)$, $R(t)$, $D(t)$ from eqs. (3.1) (for each of the 51 output points).
- The solution is displayed for t=0,52*10/50=10.4,..., 52 as programmed in Listings 1.1, 4.1 (every tenth value of t is displayed).
- ICs (1.2) are confirmed ($t = 0$), as scaled by S_{tot}.
- $S(t), Ia(t), Is(t), R(t), D(t)$ sum to a near constant value in t, starting with $S(t = 0) = 3.3 \times 10^8$. This is an important test of eqs. (3.1), (4.1) as discussed in the chapter Appendix A1.
- The deaths, $D(t = 52)$, are reduced to 5.34e+02 = 534 from 5.52e+05 = 552,000 for ncase=1. Thus, the deaths are reduced by approximately 1/1000 so that the postulated vaccine/drug treatment is very effective.
- The computational effort as indicated by ncall = 84 is modest so that lsodes computed the solution to eqs. (3.1), (4.1) efficiently.

The graphical output is in Fig. 4.1.

The solutions appear to approach a steady state inferring that the response to the virus is stable.

In summary, for ncase=1,2,

```
Table 1.6, ncase=1
          t
        52.0
        S(t)            Ia(t)            Is(t)
        R(t)            D(t)             sum
```

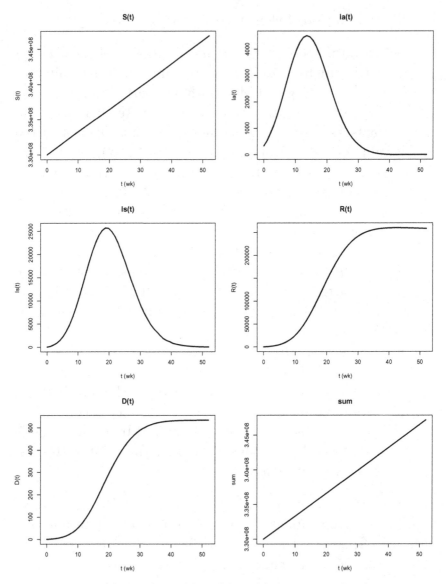

Figure 4.1: $S(t), Ia(t), Is(t), R(t), D(t)$ from eqs. (3.1), `ncase=2`

7.74e+07	2.93e+02	7.42e+04
2.69e+08	5.52e+05	3.47e+08

Table 4.1, ncase=2, kr=2

	t	
	52.0	
S(t)	Ia(t)	Is(t)
R(t)	D(t)	sum
3.47e+08	3.12e-02	3.45e+01
2.58e+05	5.34e+02	3.47e+08

The reduction by a factor of appproximately $1/1000$ of $I_a(t), I_s(t), R(t), D(t)$ at $t = 52$ is demonstrated.

In summary, k_r is a sensitive parameter in determining the final solution, that is, whether the epidemic is contained.

(4.2) Summary and conclusions

The 5×5 ODE model of Chapter 1 is extended to include a limit on the rate of transition of susceptibles to infecteds as stated in eqs. (3.1) with $rate(t)$ of eq. (4.1) (Listing 4.2). This is an example of the use of a variable coefficient in the ODE model.

If this function is interpreted as representing the introduction of a vaccine/drug, the suppression of the virus epidemic is demonstrated by comparing the solutions for **ncase=1** $(rate = 1)$ and **ncase=2** $(rate$ decreasing according to eq. (4.1)).

Chapter 5

ODE Model with Delays

(5) Introduction

The preceding analysis of eqs. (1.1), (3.1) indicates that the asymptomatic infecteds with population density $I_a(t)$ contribute significantly to the solutions $S(t)$, $I_s(t)$, $R(t)$, $D(t)$. The contribution of the asymptomatic infecteds is complicated by the incubation period (the time that symptoms are not revealed).

In the analysis that follows, the possible effect of a $I_a(t)$ delay in selected terms in eqs. (3.1) is considered.

(5.1) ODE model with delays

The rate terms in eqs. (3.1-1,2)

$$\pm r_{SI_a}(S(t) - S_{lim})I_a(t) \tag{5.1-1}$$

are modified to

$$\pm r_{SI_a}(S(t) - S_{lim})I_a(t - \tau) \tag{5.1-2}$$

The delayed $I_a(t - \tau)$ of term (5.1-2) is used in place of the contemporary $I_a(t)$ of term (5.1-1). The R routines with the delayed terms (5.1-2) are considered next.

(5.1.1) Main program

The following details pertain to the lagged term (5.1-2).

- The parameter set is defined in Listing 1.1.

```
#
# Model parameters
#
# S(t)
   rp=0.001;
   rSIa=1;
   rSIs=1;
   rR=0.001;
   Stot=3.3e+08;
   tau=2;
   ncase=1;
#
# Ia(t)
#
# Is(t)
   rIsIa=0.1;
#
# R(t)
   rRIa=0.5;
   rRIs=0.5;
#
# D(t)
   rDIa=0.001;
   rDIs=0.001;
```

Listing 5.1: Parameters for Listing 1.1

In particular, tau $= \tau$ in term (5.1-2) is defined (and used in ode1a). The original time interval is retained,

$0 \leq t \leq t_f = 52$. Two cases are programmed, `ncase=1,2` in `ode1a` as explained next.

- The R integrator for delay ODEs, `dede`, is used in place of `lsodes` (included in the R integrator library `deSolve`). The arguments `y`, `times`, `func` of `dede` are reserved names and are essentially the same as for `lsodes`. The solution of the delay ODE system is returned in matrix `out` (for subsequent display).

```
#
# Integration of delay ODEs
  out=dede(y=y0,times=tout,func=ode1a);
  nrow(out);
  ncol(out);
```

(5.1.2) ODE routine

The ODE routine `ode1a` is an extension of the routine of Listing 1.2.

```
  ode1a=function(t,y,parm,lag) {
#
# Function ode1a computes the t derivative
# vectors of S(t),Ia(t),Is(t),R(t),D(t)
#
# Delayed variables
  if (t > tau){
    ylag=lagvalue(t-tau);
  } else {
    ylag=y0; }
#
# One vector to five scalars
   S=y[1];
  Ia=y[2];
  Is=y[3];
```

```
    R=y[4];
    D=y[5];
#
# Ia(t-tau)
  if(ncase==1){Iad=Ia;}
  if(ncase==2){Iad=ylag[2];}
#
# ODEs
    St=rp-rSIa*S*Iad-rSIs*S*Is+rR*R;
    Iat=rSIa*S*Iad-rIsIa*Ia-
        rRIa*Ia-rDIa*Ia;
    Ist=rSIs*S*Is+rIsIa*Ia-
        rRIs*Is-rDIs*Is;
    Rt=rRIa*Ia+rRIs*Is-rR*R;
    Dt=rDIa*Ia+rDIs*Is;
#
# Five scalars to one vector
  yt=rep(0,5);
  yt[1]=St;
  yt[2]=Iat;
  yt[3]=Ist
  yt[4]=Rt;
  yt[5]=Dt;
#
# Increment calls to ncall
  ncall <<- ncall+1;
#
# Return ODE t vector
  return(list(c(yt)));
#
# End of ode1a
  }
```

Listing 5.2: ODE routine **ode1a** including term (5.1-2)

We can note the following details about Listing 5.2.

- A fourth argument, τ, is added, which is the delay in an ODE system [2, 1].

  ```
  ode1a=function(t,y,parm,lag) {
  ```

  In the present case, `tau` is unused, but is required in the argument list to properly interface with the delay ODE integrator, `dede` [2].
- The R utility `lagvalue` is called to delay the dependent variables in `y` (second argument of `ode1a`).

  ```
  #
  # Delayed variables
    if (t > tau){
      ylag=lagvalue(t-tau);
    } else {
      ylag=y0; }
  ```

  An `if` is used for two cases: (1) $t > \tau$ so that `lagvalue` is used to lag the ODE dependent variables (vector `y`) in t, and (2) $t \leq \tau$ for which the initial condition vector `y0` is used as the history vector of the delayed ODEs [1].
- For `ncase=1`, a delay is not added to $I_a(t)$ and the solution is then the same as in Table 1.6, Fig. 1.1 (`lsodes` and `dede` return the same solution with no delay). For `ncase=2`, $I_a(t - \tau)$ of term (5.1-2) is placed in `Iad` (the second element of `ylag`).

  ```
  #
  # Ia(t-tau)
    if(ncase==1){Iad=Ia;}
    if(ncase==2){Iad=ylag[2];}
  ```

- `Iad` is used in the rate `rSIa*(S-Slim)*Iad` of eqs. (3.1-1,2) to account for the incubation time of $I_a(t)$.

```
#
# ODEs
  St=rp-rSIa*S*Iad-rSIs*S*Is+rR*R;
  Iat=rSIa*S*Iad-rIsIa*Ia-
      rRIa*Ia-rDIa*Ia;
```

Iad could be used in other places in the programming of
the ODE system of eqs. (3.1),

• The programming of eqs. (3.1-3,4,5) remains unchanged.

The output from Listings 5.1, 5.2 follows.

(5.1.3) Numerical, graphical output

The output for ncase=2 (set in Listing 5.1) follows.

[1] 51

[1] 6

t		
0.0		
S(t)	Ia(t)	Is(t)
R(t)	D(t)	sum
3.30e+08	3.30e+02	3.30e+01
0.00e+00	0.00e+00	3.30e+08

t		
10.4		
S(t)	Ia(t)	Is(t)
R(t)	D(t)	sum
3.33e+08	1.69e+03	2.58e+04
2.89e+04	5.80e+01	3.33e+08

```
          t
        20.8
        S(t)            Ia(t)           Is(t)
        R(t)            D(t)            sum
    3.26e+08        7.89e+03        5.23e+06
    5.22e+06        1.05e+04        3.37e+08


          t
        31.2
        S(t)            Ia(t)           Is(t)
        R(t)            D(t)            sum
    1.11e+08        9.43e+03        4.31e+07
    1.85e+08        3.72e+05        3.40e+08


          t
        41.6
        S(t)            Ia(t)           Is(t)
        R(t)            D(t)            sum
    7.13e+07        8.97e+02        3.00e+06
    2.69e+08        5.44e+05        3.44e+08


          t
        52.0
        S(t)            Ia(t)           Is(t)
        R(t)            D(t)            sum
    7.54e+07        7.24e+01        1.63e+05
    2.71e+08        5.54e+05        3.47e+08


ncall =   738
```

Table 5.1: Numerical output from Listings 1.1, 5.1, 5.2,
ncase=2

We can note the following details about this output.

- 51 t output points as the first dimension of the solution matrix out from dede as programmed in the main program of Listings 1.1, 5.1 (with nout=51).
- The solution matrix out returned by dede has 6 elements as a second dimension. The first element is the value of t. Elements 2 to 6 are $S(t), Ia(t), Is(t), R(t), D(t)$ from eqs. (3.1), term (5.1-2) (for each of the 51 output points).
- The solution is displayed for t=0,52*10/50=10.4,..., 52 as programmed in Listings 1.1, 5.1 (every tenth value of t is displayed).
- ICs (1.2) are confirmed $(t = 0)$, as scaled by S_{tot}.
- $S(t), Ia(t), Is(t), R(t), D(t)$ sum to a near constant value in t, starting with $S(t = 0) = 3.3 \times 10^8$. This is an important test of eqs. (3.1), term (5.1-2) as discussed in the chapter Appendix A1.
- The steady state solutions for $S(t), R(t), D(t)$ with and without the delay τ are about the same $(t = 52.0)$.

```
Table 1.6, tau=0
          t
        52.0
        S(t)            Ia(t)           Is(t)
        R(t)            D(t)            sum
     7.74e+07        2.93e+02        7.42e+04
     2.69e+08        5.52e+05        3.47e+08


Table 5.1, tau=2
          t
        52.0
        S(t)            Ia(t)           Is(t)
        R(t)            D(t)            sum
     7.54e+07        7.24e+01        1.63e+05
     2.71e+08        5.54e+05        3.47e+08
```

This result is not unexpected since the use of τ is a dynamic aspect of the ODE model that has little effect at steady state.

- The dynamic solutions are substantially different. For example, $t = 20.8$,

```
Table 1.6, tau=0
        t
      20.8
      S(t)          Ia(t)          Is(t)
      R(t)           D(t)           sum
   2.95e+08       1.74e+06       1.83e+07
   2.21e+07       4.43e+04       3.37e+08


Table 5.1, tau=2
        t
      20.8
      S(t)          Ia(t)          Is(t)
      R(t)           D(t)           sum
   3.26e+08       7.89e+03       5.23e+06
   5.22e+06       1.05e+04       3.37e+08
```

In particular, the peak value of $I_a(t)$ is substantially lower with τ included, as indicated by a comparison of $I_a(t)$ in Figs. 1.1 and 5.1.

- ncall = 738 indicates a substantial difference in computational effort between lsodes (ncall = 135) and dede.

The graphical output is in Fig. 5.1.

The solutions appear to approach a steady state inferring that the response to the virus is stable and largely unchanged with τ included.

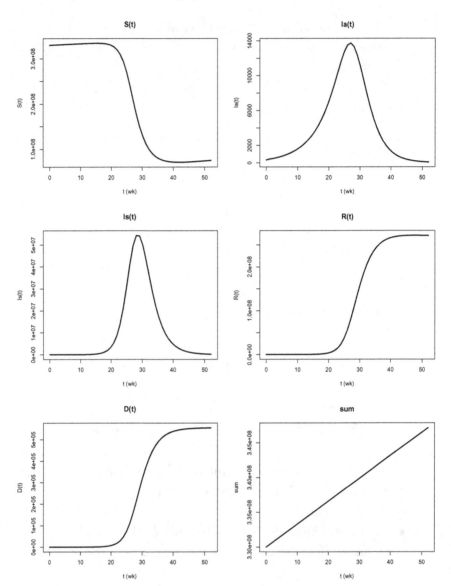

Figure 5.1: $S(t), Ia(t), Is(t), R(t), D(t)$ from eqs. (3.1) with term (5.1-2), `ncase=2`

(5.2) Summary and conclusions

The COVID-19 model incubation time for $I_a(t)$, as represented by the parameter τ in term (5.1-2), provides a significant dynamic effect, but has little effect at steady state. In particular, the recovered populations and deaths remain about the same.

The preceding example illustrates a methodology for including delayed variables in ODE models.

The ODE model with the various extensions discussed in the preceding chapters can now be used for further studies. For example,

- A sensitivity analysis of the parameters rSIa, rSIs, rDIa, rDIs so that solutions match observed deaths.
- Use of the recovereds to match the reduction in susceptibles as demonstrated by reported serous tests for antibodies.

These suggested studies are left as exercises.

References

[1] Schiesser, W.F. (2020), *Time Delay ODE/PDE Models: Applications in Biomedical Science and Engineering*, CRC press, Boca Raton, FL.

[2] Soetaert, K., J. Cash, and F. Mazzia (2012), *Solving Differential Equations in R*, Springer-Verlag, Heidelberg, Germany.

Index

A

antibodies 95
asymptomatic vii, 2–4, 8, 50
  equation 3, 20, 62
  incubation period 85

C

COVID-19 vii
  mathematical model vii–viii, 1
    asymptomatic vii, 2–4, 8, 20,
      50
    computational effort 23
    deaths vii, 3, 7, 20, 23, 29,
      58, 68–70
    delay 85, 92–93
    dependent variables vii, 2,
      19, 31
    derivative vector 18–19, 21,
      31, 35, 39, 42–59, 65
    dominant terms 46–59
    equations 1–7, 20, 62
    exponential coefficient 75
    graphical output 17, 25, 28,
      37–39, 46–59, 69, 73, 81,
      94
    incubation period 85
    infecteds vii, 1–7 *see also*
    asymptomatic,
      symptomatic

infection rate 61, 75
initial conditions vii, 8, 10,
  14
logistic rate 62, 65–66, 75, 79
main program 9, 31, 63, 87
nonlinear terms 3, 5–6, 18
  see also logistic
numerical integration vii, 10
  see also R, lsodes, dede
numerical output 16, 22, 26,
  66, 71, 79, 90
ODE routine 9, 13, 18–19,
  64–65, 77, 87, 89
parameters 9–10, 13, 24, 39,
  61–63, 70, 76, 86
programming viii, 9, 13,
  18–19
R coding viii, 9, 13, 18–19
rate constant 2, 4–8, 24, 26,
  28, 75
rate terms 3–8, 31, 37, 42, 75
recovereds vii, 1, 6, 20, 55
susceptibles vii, 1–6, 20, 47
symptomatic vii, 2–5, 8, 20,
  52
therapeutic drug viii, 29, 75,
  81
time interval 10, 14, 64, 68,
  70

time variable coefficient 75, 77
transmission rate 28–29, 75
vaccine viii, 29, 75, 81
epidemic vii–viii, 29
spatial variation vii, 1
transmission viii
rate 28–29, 75
United States vii, 1, 13

D

deaths vii, 3, 23, 58, 71, 74
equation 7, 20, 62
reduction 29, 39, 68–70, 81–83
delay 85, 92–93 *see also* R, `dede`
history vector 87
programming 87
dependent variables vii, 2, 19, 31
derivative vector 18–19, 21, 31, 35, 39, 42–59, 66
dominant terms 46–59

E

epidemic vii–viii, 29
limitation 29, 61–63 *see also* logistic
equilibrium 74, 92
exponential coefficient 75

H

history vector 87

I

incubation period 85
infecteds vii, 1–8
asymptomatic vii, 2–4, 8, 20, 50
symptomatic vii, 2–5, 8, 20, 52
infection rate
limited 61, 75
logistic 62–63, 65–66

initial condition vii, 8, 10, 14
history vector 87

L

limited infection rate 61, 75
logistic transmission rate 62
equations 62
exponential modification 75, 79
output 66, 69, 73
parameters 63
programming 65–66

M

mathematical model vii *see also* COVID-19

N

nonlinear 3, 5–6, 18
logistic 62

O

ODE
dependent variable vii, 2, 19, 31
delay 85, 92–93
history vector 87
output 90
programming 87
derivative vector 18–19, 21, 31, 35, 39, 42–44, 65
detailed analysis 31, 37, 42–59
dominant terms 46–59
equation 1–7, 20, 62
exponential coefficient 75
initial condition vii, 8, 10, 14
mathematical model vii
see also COVID-19
numerical integration vii–viii, 10
see also R, `dede`, `lsodes`
programming 18
R routine viii, 9, 13–14, 18
arguments 18

logistic rate 62, 75
terms 3
    detailed analysis 31, 37,
      42–59
    dominant 46–59
    time variable coefficient 75,
      77
ordinary differential equation *see*
ODE

P

pandemic 1
parameters 9–10, 13, 24, 39, 61–63,
    70, 76, 86
    sensitivity analysis 95

R

R scientific computing system
    application viii, 8
    availability viii
    [] matrix subscripting 10, 14
    % number format 11
      e 11
      f 11
    # comment 9
    c numerical vector 11, 17–18,
      21, 44, 52
    \n new line 11
    <<- return 18, 21
    cat 11
    dede 87, 92–93
      history vector 87
      arguments 87
    deSolve 9, 13
      see also dede, lsodes
    for 11, 15
    function 10
      arguments 10, 14–15, 18–19
    if else 87, 89
    lagvalue 87, 89
      ODE routine 89

legend 42, 47
library 9, 13
list 18, 21
lsodes 10, 14–15, 19
    atol 10
    func 10
    maxord 10
    ncol 10, 15, 22
    nrow 10, 15, 22
    ODE function 10, 18
    out 10, 15
    rtol 10
    sparsetype 10
    times 10
    y (IC) 10
matplot 42
matpoints 42
matrix 42
ncol 10, 15
nrow 10, 15
par 11, 17
plot 11, 17, 38
    arguments 11
return 18, 21
rm remove files 9, 13
rep 10, 15
seq 10, 14
setwd 9, 13
source 9, 13
sprintf 11
ylag 87–89
rate constant 2, 4–8, 24, 26, 28, 75
recovereds vii, 1, 6, 20, 55
    equation 6, 20, 62

S

serous test 95
SIR vii, 1, 29
    extension 29
social distancing 70
spatial variations vii
steady state 74, 92

susceptibles vii, 1–6, 47
  equation 1, 20, 62
switching time 70–71
symptomatic vii, 2–5, 8, 20, 52
  equation 20, 62

T

time interval 10, 14, 64
  expanded 68, 74
  switching 70–71
time switching 70–71
time variable coefficient 75, 77
therapeutic drug viii, 29, 75
  death reduction 81–83

time scale vii, 68
transmission rate 28–29, 75

V

vaccine viii, 29, 75
  death reduction 81–83

W

WHO 1
World Health Organization *see*
  WHO